Sixteen Minutes
to a Better 9-to-5

Sixteen Minutes to a Better 9-to-5

Stress-free Work with Yoga and Ayurveda

Dr. Vinod Verma

SAMUEL WEISER, INC.

York Beach, Maine

First published in 1999 by
Samuel Weiser, Inc.
P. O. Box 612
York Beach, ME 03910-0612
www.weiserbooks.com

Library of Congress Cataloging-in-Publication Data

Verma, Vinod.
    Sixteen minutes to a better 9-to-5 / Vinod Verma.
      p. cm.
    Includes bibliographical references and index.
    ISBN 1-57863-129-7 (pbk. : alk. paper)
    1. Stress management. 2. Job stress—Prevention. 3. Medicine,
Ayurvedic. 4. Yoga, Hatha. I. Title.
    RA785.V474 1999
    155.9'042—dc21   99-28896
                                             CIP

EB

Typeset in 11 point Baskerville

Cover art by Eris Klein © 1999

Printed in the United States of America

08   07   06   05   04   03   02   01   00   99
10   9   8   7   6   5   4   3   2   1

The paper used in this publication meets the minimum requirements
of the American National Standard for Permanence of Paper for
Printed Library Materials Z39.48–1984.

This book is dedicated to my paternal grandmother, who was blessed with Ayurvedic wisdom. She was a gifted healer.

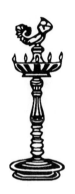

NOTE TO THE READER

The information provided in this book is not intended to replace the service of a physician. The material is presented for educational purposes, for self-help relating to health care, and for better efficiency at work. The author and the publishers are in no way responsible for any medical claims for the material presented here. To use the herbal or other remedial formulas commercially will require permission from the author.

TABLE OF CONTENTS

Principles of holistic health; Cosmic unity, and the basic
human constitution; Characteristics of the three humors—vata, pitta, and kapha; Three qualities of mind—
rajas, tamas, and sattva; Holistic health; Relationship
between work and six-dimensional human existence.

Health and non-health; Three-dimensional therapy of
Ayurveda; The "here and now" principle; Knowing body
and mind; Prakriti—your constitution; Diagnosis and
care; Revitalizing with yoga; Keeping the six-
dimensional balance.

Panchakarma, the five purification practices; Panchakarma to saptakarma; Saptakarma—seven purification
practices; Purification of the head region (nasyakarma);
Purification of the urinary tract; Saptakarma and time.

Yoga at work; General instructions for yoga practice;
The 16-minutes-a-day program; Prostration to the Sun;
Controlling the mind; Executing the 16-minute program; Priorities for the 16-minute program; Balancing
stress; Yoga for balance; Maintaining equilibrium; Yoga
activities at work; Developing a harmonious relationship with your work.

PREFACE

Two thousand six hundred years ago, Charaka, the great sage of Ayurveda, wrote the following:

> A person . . . for well-being here and in the world hereafter, should pursue three desires, such as the desire for life, the desire for wealth, and the desire for the other world. Out of all these desires, one should follow the desire to live first. Why? Because on departure from life, everything departs. Next to life, wealth should be sought, as there is nothing more sinful than to have a long life without means (of subsistence). Hence, one should make an effort to achieve means from professions, such as agriculture, animal husbandry, trade, commerce, government service, or other such noble works. . . . By working in a righteous way, one lives a long life without any dishonor.[1]

We see that the ancient wisdom of Ayurveda took into account the importance of work and the relationship of work to health and longevity. Subtracting the hours we devote to sleep, most of our waking hours are spent either at the workplace or in work-related action. It is absolutely essential to be in harmony with the atmosphere at work. If you don't like what you are doing, and if you don't get satisfaction from your chosen profession, it decelerates the work pace as well as causing health problems. Life cannot be lived in fragments. If you are unhappy with one aspect of your existence, it will affect all the other dimensions of your being. Dissatisfaction at work affects personal life; it may cause small, but nagging, ailments, or it may give rise to a serious illness in the long run.

The aim of this book is to provide a guide for building a better work atmosphere based on an understanding of Ayurvedic personality types—according to your fundamental nature or *prakriti*. It is also important to learn how to acquire a state of satisfaction in your personal life, which is essential for both better

---

[1]Charaka Samhita, Sutrasthana, XI, 4–5.

work performance and your health. Techniques used in Ayurveda and yoga will be used to help you build your own good atmosphere—even in the worst of circumstances. This is necessary today. Because of the unemployment situation all over the world, it is not so easy to change jobs or the type of work you do. When you compound the ill effects of a "bad" working situation because you are frustrated, or because you don't like what you do, you may forget why you are working in the first place, and you may affect your health. This book provides guidance to deal with these problems effectively and efficiently.

I have put forward the fundamentals of the holistic system of Ayurveda, and have provided a brief program for a holistic way of living, leading to more physical energy, freedom from small nagging ailments, more efficiency at work, a stress-free life and a state of harmony with your surroundings. These holistic principles will help you understand yourself better and you will also be able to comprehend others in a larger reference frame. This leads to more tolerance and eventually more productivity. I also focus on developing mental concentration and enhancing memory. This program is especially designed to deal with the time constraints of today's modern life-style.

Timely management of your life can save you from many health hazards and mental anguish. Investing 16 minutes every day, and few days twice a year, can prove to be an extremely profitable deal—and a source of abundant energy. Would not you be tempted to include this in your schedule?

The fundamental reason for a lack of work efficiency, fatigue, and ultimately illness, is due to the lack of maintaining your physical and mental self. With the constant use of your senses, body, and mind in this noisy and polluted world, you gradually accumulate all kinds of what I call "dirt." A regular cleaning and purification of both body and mind are suggested in the programs I present. These help enhance a feeling of well-being, which in turn means you work more effectively, which winds up being a long-term investment in your health.

By knowing the Ayurvedic personality of your colleagues—a combination of their physical conditions as well as their mental processes—you are able to know them better in terms of their functional capabilities and general reactions to life. This understanding might help you give necessary concessions to others, because you now understand their slow pace at work, or their need to be type "A" personalities. In fact, by attending group seminars on Ayurveda, people begin to understand their own reactions and this leads to a better understanding of others as well. You can improve your weak points and also experience a sense of cooperation and compassion for others. You can stop criticizing others for being too slow or too fast, and discuss these problems openly in terms of the humoral nature or fundamental constitution. You can help each other to get over your weaknesses and the work atmosphere will turn out to be like an Ayurvedic family. This can be further enhanced by doing funny exercises for relaxation—like laughing exercises or something similar during breaks. I have already tried these methods in various organizations and groups. After just one week of working together, a considerable difference was noticed in the atmosphere, and people felt more relaxed. It is obvious that when you feel relaxed and tension-free, you will be able to work better.

It will turn out to be profitable for any business to invest some money in this direction in order to make their work force stronger. After an initial practical training, it is easy to use the practices given in this book to get rid of stress and tension both at work and at home.

Dr. V. Verma
Noida/Freiburg

ACKNOWLEDGMENTS

I am extremely grateful to all my students and the people I interviewed both East and West, who very openly shared with me the pains and perils of their work situations and their personal lives. Without this insight, it would not have been possible to deal with this theme.

My special thanks to my two friends Anuroop Singh (Tony) and Heinrich Heyne, both senior executives in Delhi and Frankfurt respectively, for providing me insight into the problems of management. Tony invited me to do seminars on stress management for managers and executives, and arranged interviews with his colleagues. Inspiring discussions with Heinrich made me put this book on the priority list and his lucid views were always of great help.

My Ayurvedic guru (guide and mentor) Professor Priya Vrat Sharma appreciated my treating this theme related to work efficiency, and provided constant inspiration and guidance. He helped me become a medium for spreading Ayurvedic wisdom in the world. I express my tremendous gratitude and feel honored to be his pupil.

For the photographs, I am grateful to my brother Kuldeep (Kuku), Rajesh (Ruby), my nieces Gayatri and Shruti, and nephew Abhinav.

1

HOLISTIC HEALTH—
A JOURNEY FROM INNER TO OUTER

IT IS ESSENTIAL to understand the fundamental approach of Ayurveda before applying its practical aspects in daily life. Our modern Western approach to life is fragmented; we have compartmentalized the various aspects of human existence. Let's look at a holistic view of life and health, for this outlook is fundamental to the Ayurvedic approach.

PRINCIPLES OF HOLISTIC HEALTH

The principles of holistic health are based upon a fundamental cosmic unity. The cosmos is a dynamic whole, where everything is constantly changing; nothing happens without reason or by chance, and everything has a purpose and a goal. Health may be defined as a state of harmony within yourself and with your surroundings. Ill health or disease is caused when your being is no longer in harmony with the cosmic order. You, as an individual, are a part of this dynamic cosmos, and in order to maintain good health, you have to make an effort to keep yourself in tune with the cosmic orchestra. In simple terms, you have to adopt a way of living that is in harmony with fundamental cosmic principles. You, as an individual, are an indivisible unity, who cannot be reduced in terms of your parts, nor can you be regarded as an independent entity from the rest of the cosmos.

The modern approach to health care is based upon different principles however, and contrary to the holistic one, it is completely fragmented. The human body is compared to a machine that can be analyzed in terms of its parts. An illness is viewed as the malfunctioning of a part of the body-machine. The various mechanisms of the body are understood at biological and molecular levels, and for the purpose of treatment, body and mind are considered as separate entities. Chance plays an important role in the transformation from a healthy to an unhealthy state.

According to the modern Western medical system, all human beings are considered alike. From the Ayurvedic point of view, human beings are ever-changing, dynamic beings—like the rest of nature. They are variable in their fundamental constitution or *prakriti* (which means physical reactions as well as personality).

The holistic concept of health is very broad based. Even if you consider yourself healthy, because the mechanisms of your body function well, you still may be unhealthy if you are often dissatisfied, get angry easily, feel irritated or restless, do not sleep well, do not evacuate with ease, yawn too much, or hiccup frequently, etc.

During recent years some disastrous events on our globe have led us to review the fragmented approach of modern science. Holes in the ozone layer, the atomic leak at Chernobyl, war in the Gulf, have made us realize how far-reaching are the effects of these global events. These incidents are directly related to human health and will affect generations to come.

Imagine the cosmic reality in terms of a spiral (fig. 1). Your physical self is the innermost part of the spiral.[1] Then comes the reality of your immediate surroundings, like your family, or near and dear ones. This is followed by your social surroundings, place of work and the day-to-day interaction with the outer world. Next to this are your larger environments, such as your country and your global environment. This latter is followed by the cosmic environment. Thus, the multiple layers of reality which unfold into each other are interconnected, interrelated, and interdependent.

---

[1] In the context of Ayurvedic or Indian tradition, the physical self refers to both body and mind. In fact, it is distinguished from "soul," which is energy, and is the cause of consciousness. Body and mind are not considered independent of each other as all the physical and mental functions coordinate with each other and are interconnected and interdependent.

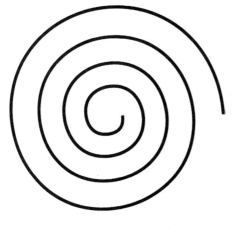

Figure 1. Cosmic reality in terms of a spiral.

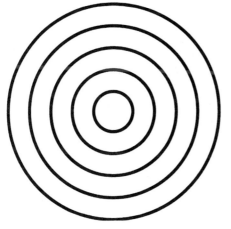

Figure 2. The closed circles within each other show that the cosmic reality is not in fragments where various dimensions of existence enclose each other in the form of independent circles.

Each cell of your body is a world by itself. It can build, construct, ingest, destroy, and do much more. The cells are grouped together to make organisms. Cells in an organism perform a coordinated function and work in harmony with each other for the fulfillment of a goal. Various organisms of the body work in harmony with each other and perform all functions of your living being. Each smaller organization is within another equally perfected bigger organization, yet the bigger ones do not enclose the smaller ones (fig. 2). Instead, the bigger emerges out of the smaller, or the smaller terminates into the bigger one forming a

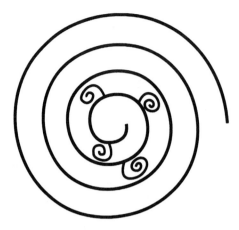

Figure 3. The development of sub-systems in the spiral reality.

spiral (fig. 1). This way, the whole cosmic reality is formed. The smaller, the bigger, and the still bigger are connected to each other in continuum in such a way that disturbance in one causes disturbance in all.

Now, let us see how an ailment is caused in this perfectly ordered, harmonious system. In the context of health, your physical body is an "organization" established within a given order and in a certain balance between the natural forces of creation and destruction. When the balance is upset, the normal rhythm of the spiral is disturbed. This gives rise to the development of one or several subsystems, which results in chaos, as the subsystems are not in harmony with the cosmic organization (fig. 3). If this chaos is left unattended at the initial stages, the subsystems grow bigger and bigger, and challenge the existence of your physical organization. The energy and activity of the body is directed to nourish the subsystem and slowly the whole being gets out of tune with cosmic harmony. This is what a major disease is.

The role of Ayurveda, or any other truly holistic system of health care, is to maintain the natural harmony of the body in order to keep it in tune with the rest of the universe. In case of an ailment, its role is to intervene early enough to stop the development of the subsystems and restore the bodily rhythm again.

At the initial stages, the pathological materials are transitory and simple practices can help restore the natural balance. The state of health in Ayurveda is called *prakriti* (nature or natural harmony in the human constitution) and the state of non-health or disease is called *vikriti* (diversion from natural harmony). The role of the physician is to restore the natural balance by intervening in the pathological cycle and starting the healthy processes again with the help of appropriate diet and drugs. Drugs are used to help nature to regain the lost harmony.[2] The Ayurvedic sages said that the cure is effected by nature itself, the physician and the drug only assist in the process. For example, a man may slip and fall and may get up by himself after some time, but if he is given support by someone, he will be able to get up in a shorter time and with less difficulty.[3]

COSMIC UNITY AND
THE BASIC HUMAN CONSTITUTION

The material reality of the whole universe is made of five basic elements—ether, air, fire, water, and earth. These five elements are organized in a variety of forms, shapes, and proportions that account for the diversity of our phenomenal world. The cause of consciousness, or vitality, or life is, however, an indestructible and immutable form of energy. Figure 4 (page 6) shows an individual's physical reality using a triangle. The point at the center represents the energy that breathes life into matter.

The five elements constitute the universal reality at various levels. Their equilibrium in the cosmos speaks for harmony and balance, whereas their vitiation causes catastrophes. For example, the life-giving wind is catastrophic in the form of a hurricane. An earthquake can bring awful destruction in seconds. The calm beautiful river that sustains life can bring another series of catastrophes. Sun makes life possible on our planet, but an excessively hot summer leads to drought and the destruction of our crops.

---

[2]P. V. Sharma, (1994). "Ayurveda moves with Nature," in *NAMAH* (*New Approaches to Medicine and Health*), vol. 1, Issue 2, (Pondicherry: Sri Aurobindo Society).
[3]Charaka Samhita, Sutrasthana, X, 5.

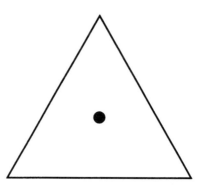

Figure 4. Symbolic representation of the physical and spiritual being of an individual.

The same cosmic principles are applied to the human body. The five elements that constitute the body are represented in the form of the three humors (or vital forces) which are responsible for all the physical and mental functions of the body. These humors are vata, pitta, and kapha. Vata is derived from ether and air, pitta from fire, and kapha from water and earth.

Vata, like the basic elements it is derived from, is all-pervasive and mobile. It is also light, subtle, cold, dry, and rough. It is responsible for all those functions which are associated with motion and which are everywhere in the body. That includes all physical movement and mind activities—blood circulation, respiration, excretion, speech, sensation, touch, hearing, feelings (such as fear, anxiety, grief, enthusiasm, etc.), natural urges, the formation of the fetus, the sexual act, and retention.

Pitta is hot—like the basic element from which it is derived. It is also characteristic of being sharp, sour, pungent, and has a fleshy smell. It is responsible for vision, digestion, hunger, thirst, heat regulation, softness, luster, cheerfulness, intellect, and sexual vigor.

Kapha is derived from the basic elements of earth and water, and like these elements, it is soft, solid, dull, sweet, heavy, cold, slimy, unctuous, and immobile. It constitutes all the solid structure of the body, and is responsible for binding, firmness, heaviness, strength, forbearance, restraint, and sexual potency.

When these three humors are in balance individually and with respect to each other, they denote a state of good health. However, if there is a disturbance in one humor and it deviates from its quantity, quality, and place, or if the three humors are not in proportion to each other, it leads to *vikriti,* or a state of impairment, thus giving rise to various ailments.

Each person has a different "basic constitution" due to various proportions and combinations of the three fundamental forms of vitality (vata, pitta, and kapha). For example, one may have a vata, or pitta, or kapha constitution. This means that one humor dominates the body. The basic constitution may be even more complicated than that, for two humors may dominate simultaneously. Vata-pitta, vata-kapha, kapha-pitta are three more types of constitutions. The seventh constitution is one where all three humors are in equal balance, creating yet a different body type.

Many variations in the efficiency, intelligence, intellect, and general energy level among the people around us also help us understand how very individual we are.

The third variant in the basic constitution is the degree of domination in the first six types of constitutions. For example, a person may have a slight vata-dominating tendency or an excessive vata-dominating tendency. Thus, we find that there are many variations in individual constitutions. In order to maintain good health and enhance your lifespan, it is important to keep your particular constitution in balance.

Before we go into the details of each humor, it is essential to understand that they are not static. The cosmos is a dynamic whole, and like anything else, the humors alter with time, space, nutrition, and other activities. If they were static, then the whole scientific basis of making a personal effort to maintain an equilibrium would be lost. The basis of Ayurveda is that you are like gardeners of your own destiny, and through your personal effort, you can work for good health—or ruin it completely.[4]

---

[4]According to Ayurveda, the circumstances (relating to health or otherwise) over which we have no control are the results of deeds or karma from previous lives, and are termed *daiva.* All effort made in this life is called *purushakara.* For good health and longevity, there must be a coordination between *daiva* and *purushakara.* It means that we are provided with certain terrain and we have to work on it according to its basic quality in order to get the best results. With our *purushakara* (personal effort), we can build a palace from ruins, and we can also turn a palace into ruins. In other words, even if we are blessed with good health, we must make a constant effort to maintain it as everything is constantly changing in this universe. (See Charaka Samhita, Vimanasthanam, III, 29–35).

Since everything in the universe is made of the same five basic elements, everything around us affects us in terms of our humoral balance. A glass of water, a pinch of salt, weather, climate, the time of the day, the geographical location, etc. Everything that helps establish balance is a medicine, and everything that disturbs this balance is poisonous. For example, on a hot summer day, you may have pain in your feet and legs due to excessive sweating. A glass of cold water with lemon and some salt will cure this pain by reestablishing the body's balance. However, the same drink taken on a winter evening may do harm by enhancing vata and pitta, and it will make the body hold too much water. Cold sweetened milk helps cure heartburn and the side-effects of excessively spicy food. However, the same cold milk may harm someone suffering from heaviness and a cold sensation in the body. These latter are the signs of disturbed kapha, and cold milk enhances the humor further as it is also kapha-dominating, and does more harm than good in this particular case. The medicine in Ayurveda is given according to the individual constitution after taking into account the place and time. All this will be more clear after we have gone through the details of each humor, signs of its domination, factors that affect it, signs of vitiation, and its treatment.

CHARACTERISTICS OF THE THREE HUMORS

Vata Domination

Imagine that you are attending a class with twenty other students, and the teacher needs something. The first one to get up is the vata type. The one first to answer the telephone in a group or family will also come in this category as far as the basic constitution is concerned. Vata-dominating people are agile, quick, swift to act, unrestricted in their movements, enthusiastic, quick to respond emotionally (fear and anxiety), and are easily irritated. They are intolerant to cold, and shiver easily. They have coarse hair and nails, and have unusually prominent blood vessels. Depending upon the degree of vata domination, you may have these characteristics in varying degrees and may not have all of them.

Factors that Disturb Vata: Let's see which factors vitiate vata so that vata-dominating people can avoid them. Fasting, delaying meals, and staying hungry will disturb the vital functions of this humor. Keeping awake late at night, exposure to cold wind, eating over-ripe dry food and food that is preserved after preparation (*basa*)[5] are some additional factors that will disturb this humor further. The rainy season, evening, last part of the night, old age, forest and mountain climates are also vata-dominating. Injury and blood loss disturbs vata and so does bad posture or sleeping on hard surfaces. Leading a hectic life-style, and dealing with emotions such as guilt, fear, and anxiety contribute to disturb vata. Excessive indulgence in sexual intercourse also leads to vata vitiation.

It is obvious that a vata-dominant person will be more easily affected by all that tends to vitiate this humor. First of all, you must know what the symptoms are and what therapeutic measures must be taken to regain balance.

Signs of Vitiated Vata: If you get up in the morning with a stiff body, often have bad taste in your mouth, and suffer from a dry throat and mouth, this humor is certainly impaired. That means that your vata is diverted from its normal and natural path (prakriti) and is undergoing deformation (vikriti).

Vitiation of vata may also lead to a general fatigue, stomach ache, dry skin, dark colored stool, giddiness, tremors, yawning, hiccups, malaise, and delirium. It may give rise to dry skin, a dull complexion, pain in the temporal region, insomnia, and withdrawn or timid behavior. One or more of these symptoms confirm that the person is suffering from vata impairment and should immediately attend to it by avoiding everything that leads to the vitiation of this humor and taking some therapeutic measures.

Curing Vitiated Vata: For curing imbalanced vata, you need to eat sweet, sour, or hot foods, and should avoid salty and dry nutrition. Hot baths, a Turkish bath, and any other means of heat applications to the body should be used. You could take an

---

[5]*Basa* is a term applied to food that is kept for several hours after preparation. For example, food prepared early in the morning will be basa by evening. All forms of preserved foods are technically basa and tend to disturb vata functions in the body.

enema with vata-decreasing drugs. Anointing your body with hot oils, or getting a massage is very valuable to cure the pathological effects of this vitiation. Appropriate rest, relaxation, sleep, a peaceful atmosphere, and a cheerful mental state are other measures that are important.

Pitta Domination

People who are intolerant of heat and who usually have a hot face and lustrous complexion are pitta-dominant. The people in this category usually have a tendency to moles, freckles, or pimples, have excessive hunger and thirst, and have strong body odor. They are generally intolerant and lack endurance. They tend to lose their hair or go gray rather early.

Factors that Disturb Pitta: Eating excessively spicy, hot (chilies, etc.), or salty foods, or drinking alcohol or eating foods that give you a burning sensation will impair this humor. Midnight and noon are the pitta-dominating times, while the desert and coastal regions are the pitta-dominating places. Excessive sun bathing may diminish pitta and autumn (the equivalent to summer in Europe) is the pitta season, whereas youth is the pitta time of life. Excess anger can also lead to the vitiation of this humor.

Signs of Vitiated Pitta: When pitta no longer functions normally, you may feel abnormally hungry or thirsty. You may perspire excessively, or have strong body odor, or you may suffer from a tearing and thickening of the skin. Rashes, acne, and herpes are some other signs of pitta vikriti. Burning sensations and excessive heat in the body may be experienced, and you may constantly have a feeling of dissatisfaction and anger.

Curing Vitiated Pitta: The best therapeutic measure for treating vitiated pitta is to take bitter, sweet, astringent, or cold foods. Cold baths and massage, or pasting the body with cooling things (like sandalwood paste or mud) are some of the very effective measures to treat this vitiation. Drugs with purgative qualities are used to get rid of this vitiation. Consolation and emotional support are additional therapeutic measures in this direction.

Kapha Domination

Kapha-dominant people are usually exactly the opposite of vata-dominant people, as they are rather slow in their activities and do not tend to take the initiative. They take time to make decisions. They are generally stable in their movements and have strong bodies. Opposite to the pitta type, they have little hunger, thirst, or perspiration. They have clear eyes and a clear complexion.

Factors that Disturb Kapha: Excessively salty, oily, or fatty foods, a sedentary life-style, lack of exercise, and daydreaming lead to the vitiation of this humor. Childhood, the spring season, the first part of the night, and the early morning are the times when you tend to suffer from the imbalance of this humor.

Signs of Vitiated Kapha: Kapha imbalance gives rise to a constant feeling of drowsiness, and you tend to sleep excessively. Fatigue caused by kapha impairment is different from that of vata, as in the former you have heaviness in the body, and in the latter you feel stiff. Vata fatigue is cured by rest, whereas kapha fatigue increases with rest. If your kapha is vitiated, the more you sleep, the more you feel drowsy. A sweet taste in the mouth and excessive salivation are further signs of vitiated kapha. Kapha vitiation may give rise to nausea, an itchy feeling in the throat, whiteness in the urine, eyes, and feces. Weariness, lassitude, and depression are further signs of kapha problems.

Curing Vitiated Kapha: You should eat pungent, bitter, astringent, and sharp foods. Wet heat is helpful. You must force yourself to be active, to sleep less, and to do plenty of physical exercise to get back the balance in this humor. Emesis or forced vomiting is one of the purification practices done to reestablish the balance.

After having reviewed the basics of the three vital forces that control all the functions of body and mind, it is clear that when they are not in balance, we suffer from physical ailments. In addition, this disharmony leads to mental and personality problems. For example, a person with diminished vata may be too frantic, may not listen to others properly, and may cause problems at work because he or she is acting like an egg-beater. Similarly, the one with vitiated pitta may disturb the atmosphere with fits of anger and intolerant behavior—especially at noon time, before lunch. The one with kapha problems may be too slow and inefficient. Thus, to some extent, we are driven to certain actions by the three vital forces when they are not in harmony within our body. Our quest for balance begins from a very basic, physical level of existence, and the journey continues to embrace the larger aspect of reality—the mind.

THREE QUALITIES OF MIND—RAJAS, TAMAS, AND SATTVA

Just as vata, pitta, and kapha are the three major forces working at the physical level, the mind also has three kinds of functional qualities which should maintain balance for your well-being. These are activity (*rajas*), inactivity (*tamas*), and stillness (*sattva*). Thinking, planning, and making decisions are rajas qualities of the mind. We can say that a normal working day is rajas-dominant. While you sleep, your mind is closed to any new knowledge; the senses withdraw temporarily from their activities, and this state is qualified as tamas. Qualities, such as greed, jealousy, laziness, pain, and killing, etc., which hinder the expansion of the mind, are also in the tamas category. Sattva qualities of the mind are those which lead toward balance, stillness, goodness, truth, compassion, and virtue. These are qualities that are developed through self-discipline, self-restraint, control over the senses, controlled breathing, yogic postures, and single-pointedness of the mind. (Though technically wrong, the single-pointedness of the mind, or dhyana, is called "meditation" in common parlance. For more details on this theme, refer to my book, *Yogasutras of Patanjali.*)[6]

---

[6] V. Verma, (1996) *Yogasutras of Patanjali: A Scientific Exposition* (New Delhi: Clarion Books).

The imbalance of these three qualities of mind lead to a large number of ailments. Life in technologically advanced industrialized nations is rajas- and tamas-dominant, and there is no place or time for sattva. This leads to insomnia, hypertension, and various mental disorders. Greed, dissatisfaction, and excessive attachment to material possessions are major characteristics that take away the peace of humanity. Fortunately, all over the world, we have realized that, and there is now a move to revive sattva activities—to initiate stillness of the mind—meditation.

According to Ayurveda, the **first priority** of life should be safeguarding health because when you are ill, nothing matters. The **second priority** is earning enough money to live, because a long life is miserable without the appropriate means of survival. After having fulfilled these two basic needs, the **third priority** is spiritual fulfillment. The second priority seems to be the major concern of people in our times and they end up caught in its web. By creating a balance between the three qualities of mind by implementing some simple daily practices, you can manage to get out of this web.

A hectic day, full of activities and meetings with various people gives rise to extremely fast mental activity. After such a day, it may be possible that you have difficulty sleeping, or you may not sleep peacefully. However, if you take some time for yourself—to be still, to meditate—after work and before you go to bed, your sleep can be rejuvenating, and you may wake up full of energy the next day.

The three vital functions of the body on the physical plane and the three activities of the mind are interconnected and interdependent. For example, someone who has been working at a hectic pace all day, who has been working under a lot of pressure (an excess of rajas), who then has problems sleeping may slowly develop a vata impairment. This person may begin to suffer from constipation, nervousness, hypertension, or other symptoms related to vata functions. Similarly, an imbalance of vata, which may initially develop from an inappropriate diet, may slowly lead to a hectic mental state, nervousness, and sleep disorders. A lack of self-control and outbursts of anger (tamas) may lead to pitta impairment. A vitiated pitta caused by the wrong diet (like too much sour food or alcohol) may make one easily angry and intolerant.

Similarly, a person with impaired kapha may slowly fall into a depression because of inactivity and too much sleep. On the other hand, a person dealing with depression due to excessive tamas activity in the mind may begin to suffer from disorders due to kapha vitiation. Since one factor effects the other, one gets into a vicious cycle of events. At this stage, one needs to work with one's body, mind, and vitality (soul) *simultaneously* by applying Ayurvedic three-dimensional therapy, which is explained in the next chapter.

HOLISTIC HEALTH

The essence of holistic health is to create a balance between the six different vital forces of human existence—three at the physical level and three at the mental level. These two categories of three each cannot be separated because they are interconnected and interdependent. At the physical level, if one humor vitiates, it slowly diminishes the others as they work in cooperation with each other. For example, if vata is diminished, it will disturb the functions of pitta, just as a flame cannot withstand too much wind. Vitiation of kapha in certain parts of the body will block the passage of vata and will cause other problems.

Figures 5 and 6 are representations of the connection between the six vital forces at various physical and mental levels. Figure 5 represents the connection of vata to rajas, pitta to sattva, and kapha to tamas. Vata and rajas are both related to movement and action. The qualities of sattva are purity, truthfulness, compassion, and virtue, and are represented by light. These qualities enlighten your mind. Pitta represents physical fire and energy. Kapha is the vital force that creates the physical body and thus it renders form and provides a corpus for the other two vital forces. At the mental level, tamas represents inaction and inertia. Action cannot exist without inaction; truth and virtue are valued because the qualities opposing them exist. Figure 6 represents the second aspect of the interrelationship and interdependence of these six vital forces. Visualize the two triangles of the three humors and three qualities moving constantly along the same axis. The present position represents the ideal state of balance and harmony.

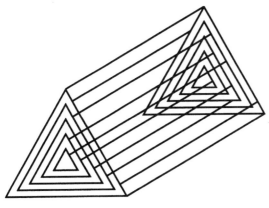

Figure 5. The interrelationship between the three humors (vata, pitta, kapha) and the three qualities of the mind (rajas, sattva, tamas) at various levels of existence.

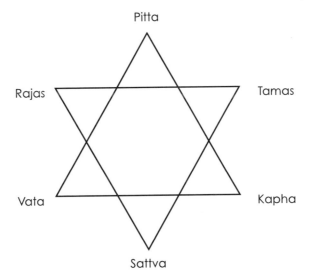

Figure 6. The six dimensional human existence and an ideal state of balance and harmony.

RELATIONSHIP BETWEEN WORK AND
SIX-DIMENSIONAL HUMAN EXISTENCE

To create a harmonious and peaceful atmosphere at any social level or work environment, we have to consider the people who form the group. In a healthy body, all the parts are in rhythm with nature, and in a group there has to be a balanced physical and mental level in order to create a coordinated social rhythm. Ayurvedic principles are easy to apply and they help us enhance our physical and mental capabilities and our social potential.

Ayurveda does not segregate the various aspects of an individual's existence. We know that our health problems affect the personality and vice versa. Similarly, problems and clashes at work often have their roots in our health and private life. These problems create a vicious cycle, and we eventually reach a state where we do not know how to begin curing the problem. Many people reach a point of exhaustion in these kinds of circumstances and end up with a serious illness. To create a balance for good health and harmony, Ayurveda suggests that we lead a wholesome life. For this it is also essential that we bring holistic values to our work arena. It is not possible to maintain balance in our lives with respect to the six dimensions described earlier if we only make an effort at the familial and individual levels, especially if we spend eight or nine hours unpleasantly at work. Ultimately, the substantial part of our day will dominate the rest, and we will not be able to live in harmony. Recognition of the many dimensions of human existence can lead to flexibility, understanding, and mutual cooperation at the workplace. When people at work have mutual support from each other and some common aim besides their work, they acquire happy and satisfied dispositions. This state of mind will lead to better health, an enhanced working capacity, and a reduced number of lost days caused by illness.

The following chapters explain simple methods to change your lifestyle, which, with a little investment of your time, will get you large returns at different levels of your existence.

2

PRESERVING THE
STATE OF HEALTH

THE INTRODUCTORY CHAPTER has provided you with an overall view of the holistic system of Ayurveda. Let us see how these principles apply to the individual and how you can develop the sensitivity needed in order to keep watch on your state of health.

HEALTH AND NON-HEALTH

Your state of health is not a static state. From time to time, even the healthiest of us fall prey to minor ailments, or feel unwell in one way or another. Generally, we recover and return to our state of health. Being unwell, or having a minor ailment, is temporary and I'll call it a state of "non-health." In Ayurveda the two stages of health and non-health are called *prakriti* and *vikriti* respectively. *Prakriti* means "nature," and the basic nature of the body is to stay healthy. *Prakriti* also denotes our basic constitution which I will explain in detail later. *Vikriti* means "a deviation from the natural state of health."

Many times during our lives, we will pass from the state of health to non-health and vice versa. We begin with the hypothesis that just as the state of health is not static, the state of non-health is also temporary. Our energy should be directed toward guarding our health, by preventing ourselves from falling into the state of non-health, and secondly by recovering quickly when we allow ourselves to get out of balance.

STATE OF HEALTH $\Longleftrightarrow$ STATE OF NON-HEALTH

If we let the state of non-health persist too long because we neglect caring for ourselves, the process of reversal becomes more and more difficult. The longer we delay, the longer and harder it is to heal ourselves. And, if the state of non-health is allowed to persist for years, it may reach a stage where the condition is only partially reversible. That is what a serious disease is.

Let's consider some examples to clarify the above statements. To get blisters in your mouth is a state of non-health. They can be very painful, and make one suffer during the process of chewing food. They are usually caused due to pitta vitiation. Generally, they appear during the change of season from cold to hot, or due to an inappropriate diet for the hot season. If one eats too many potatoes, garlic, cheese, nuts, pork, and other pitta-promoting foods during the hot season, and does not drink enough cold water, one may suffer from blisters, or from other pitta ailments. If, when they first appear, you change to a pitta-reducing diet (cold milk, rice, fish, carrots, papaya, figs, fennel, anise, and so on), you will be able to recover from this minor ailment very quickly. However, if you treat them externally, and keep adding fuel to the fire with a pitta diet, you will not be cured properly, and this ailment may become chronic. When the ailment becomes chronic, it will be harder to cure and the recurrence of this ailment might lead to other mouth infections in addition.

Let's look at another example of someone who suffers from constipation, which is a vata ailment. Irregular, hard, dark colored stool, or only a partial evacuation are symptoms of constipation. It is easy to cure this state of non-health by drinking hot water in the morning, taking an appropriate diet, and removing other factors which cause this ailment. However, if it is not attended to, and is allowed to persist, it gives rise to gastric trouble, headaches, fatigue, disturbed sleep, bad dreams, and giddiness. These troubles create a further imbalance of vata and may bring on other related ailments. Constipation may cause hemorrhoids (piles) or even colitis if it is not attended to for a very long time. Once there is a serious disorder, simple Ayurvedic home remedies are generally not sufficient to cure it.

Let's look at another example—the common cold. This example is slightly different from the one above as in this case the state of non-health is not directly due to the imbalance of the humors[1] but is caused by an external attack. It is an ailment related to kapha, where the mucous membrane is inflamed and an excess of mucus is formed. However, you get this cold because your life-giving forces—the three humors—are not in balance, and this diminishes the general ability of the body to fight this external attack of virus or bacteria. In this case, you need to rest and should eat a warm, pitta-enhancing, kapha-decreasing diet in order to regain your health. Cold drinks, other cold foods, sweet, salty, or oily food, and an exposure to cold will prolong the state of non-health. If the cold persists too long because of negligence, it may lead to sinus infection.[2] This latter may become chronic and may weaken the sense of sight, hearing, smell, or may cause some other allied problems. Thus, it is absolutely essential that you should make every effort to get rid of a cold quickly.

Recovery from the state of non-health to health is a natural phenomenon, but our efforts, drugs, and physicians play a role to hasten this process. The examples show that, through negligence, ignorance, or wrong treatment, we may delay the process of recovery. Therefore, appropriate knowledge about your body, consulting a good holistic physician,[3] and the right drugs are very important.

---

[1]According to Ayurveda, the diseases are classified into three categories—innate, exogenous, and psychic. Innate diseases are those which arise due to imbalances in the three humors—vata, pitta, and kapha. Exogenous diseases are those which arise due to external factors like poisons, polluted air, parasites, bacteria, virus, etc. Psychic diseases are those caused by unfulfilled desires and facing the undesired.

These three types of diseases are interdependent. A constant imbalance of the three humors not only leads to innate disorders, but also brings down the *ojas* (immunity and vitality) of the body, thus paving way for all kinds of external attacks. On the other hand, exogenous disorders disturb the humoral equilibrium and may also lead to innate diseases. Innate disorders like insomnia, nervousness (vata disorders), or lassitude and inertia (kapha disorders), may lead to various psychic ailments.

[2]In our cranium (the bones of the upper part of the head), there are many cavities, which are known as sinuses. When any of these cavities gets inflamed and infected, it is called sinusitis.

[3]A good holistic physician is one who does not treat your body like a machine, who examines you in your totality. He or she does not only focus on the ailing part, but goes to the root of the problem, and determines the factors causing the disorder. She or he should have knowledge and practical experience, and should be friendly and cheerful.

THE THREE-DIMENSIONAL THERAPY OF AYURVEDA

Up until this point we have discussed various methods of therapy for regaining our health. Ayurveda recommends three-dimensional therapy in case of an ailment. The three types are rational, psychological, and spiritual, and they should be applied simultaneously. (See figure 7.) We can also apply these principles to maintain our health, to cure minor ailments, and to prevent disease.

Rational therapy: This involves eating the right kinds of foods, allowing ourselves enough rest, doing inner cleaning practices, such as enema, emesis, purgation, etc., massage, anointing, appropriate physical exercise. It also allows for a congenial atmosphere so that we can heal, and requires that we deal with our environment—allowing for changes in weather and season.

Psychological therapy: Here we use mental effort and energy in the process of recovery. Our thought process is directed toward searching for the causes of the ailment, factors enhancing it, and we will use our will power to eradicate these conditions. In the present context, when we are talking about maintaining health, it is also possible to learn to direct mental energy to help "fix" health problems. However, when people are sick, they may not be

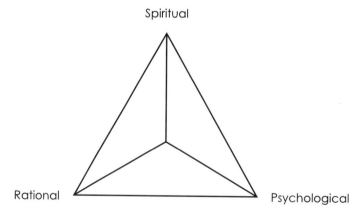

Figure 7. The three-dimensional therapy of Ayurveda.

able to direct mental energy to the process of healing. We need to seek help from some elderly wise person, or our physician may give mental support and courage so we can gradually gain strength. We can achieve this using sattva activities and various yogic and meditative practices.

Spiritual therapy: We can recite mantras, wear roots and gems, carry out auspicious acts, make offerings, follow religious precepts, fast, invoke blessings, give ourselves to the gods, make donations, take pilgrimages, and atone for our actions. Roots, seeds, gems, and so forth are used for spiritual therapy because they are known to contain specific cosmic energy. Carrying them influences the body's subtle energy. Blessed objects from holy places and from holy persons, prayers, pilgrimages, and worship, contain cosmic power beyond our material reality and may help us establish a connection with the limitless, timeless, and endless energy of the cosmos. The cosmic energy is used for healing and developing our mental faculties.

THE "HERE AND NOW" PRINCIPLE

According to Ayurveda, illness satiates the vital forces of life (*rasashoshana*). Thus, when the state of "non-health" persists for a long time, the general vitality diminishes and we become vulnerable to all kinds of other ailments. We should pay attention to the three major aspects of the state of non-health—the intensity, duration, and frequency—and try to reduce them. These three factors become more obvious as we grow older. That means that our capacity to recover slows down. However, if we keep our balance we can maintain youthful vigor and vitality. For that, we need to be aware of what we do. This does not mean that we need to do two hours in the gym per week, or jog every morning and evening, or eat a measured diet in terms of calories, or hundreds of other do's and don'ts. Don't be a health fanatic. Ayurveda allows you to eat and do almost anything, but it suggests a middle path. We should avoid excess, and should make nutritional combinations that will maintain the body's natural equilibrium.

KNOWING BODY AND MIND

Since most professional people do not have a lot of spare time, you need to find efficient ways to keep yourself healthy. Knowledge of mind-body and the environment will be the foundation you build on. Gradually, your knowledge will transform into wisdom and you will begin to "feel" the state of equilibrium and will not do anything that goes against it. Health care practice should be pleasurable—like a game of chess. Each move should be made intelligently, but not mechanically. Taking care of yourself should be spontaneous; it should be a part of your being, just as your instinct functions naturally. Your body is the seat of all pains and pleasure. It is the "self" with which you identify yourself. The aim of Ayurveda is to enhance pleasure and to diminish pain. You can achieve this aim by slowly adopting activities and actions that maintain a harmonious natural state of balance within yourself and your surroundings. Preserving health using painstaking methods is not recommended in Ayurveda.

The difference between the state of health and non-health is sometimes very fragile. We all go through phases when we feel unwell but the symptoms are vague. Therefore, we hesitate to seek the help of a physician and we suffer from minor but sometimes nagging health problems. I call these symptoms "subjective symptoms." It means that they are not objective as we know them from pre-existing norms. We should not ignore these insignificant subjective symptoms and should attend to them without delay. The holistic system of Ayurveda teaches us the importance and significance of these symptoms and advises us to make an effort to cure them at the initial stage. For example, according to Ayurveda, yawning (except when it is time to sleep) is a state of non-health. Excessive, untimely yawning indicates vata vitiation. By taking appropriate measures to balance vata using massage, appropriate diet, sleep and rest, we can restore the state of health.

Keeping Watch

The Ayurvedic concept of maintaining health requires that we pay attention to the balance of body and mind so that we make the right moves at the right time. We must reestablish balance as soon as it diverts from its normal path. I call this the "principle of here and now." We can observe minor diversions and mend them immediately. To stay healthy only requires that we pay attention to the messages our body sends us.

Purification

When you take a shower every day, there is very little dirt on your body. It is immediately cleaned and you feel good and fresh afterward. Imagine someone lazy and dirty who takes a bath or a shower only twice a month. Most of you will react by saying, "Sure this fellow has a lot to clean." Just as the outer parts of the body accumulate dirt every day, similarly, the inner parts of the body also accumulate dirt over a period of time and require periodic cleaning to revitalize their functions.

A constant use of the senses and the mind, the effect of various stressful and tense situations, and other excessively emotional events affect the mind. It needs periodic purification through yogic exercises, breathing practices, and concentration exercises (meditation). If cleaning and purification of the internal organs and inner self is not done, one day the "accumulated dirt" weighs heavy and it may develop a subsystem of its own (see chapter 1 for the details of subsystems and ailments). Thus, to avoid illness, and to maintain longevity, cleansing and purification practices are absolutely necessary.

A gain in an investment depends upon taking the proper action at the right time. Investment in your health can be seen in a similar manner. If a humor vitiates, or is on the verge of vitiation, you can do several things. You can find the vitiating factors and stop all those actions that have caused this diversion. When you devote your energy to pacify this vitiation immediately, the problem is solved easily. If you are negligent and do not understand the language of your body, you may not take the proper actions and you vitiate further the already disturbed humor. This will, of course, lead to one or more of the ailments related to that humor. Then you will deal with illness. It's better to stick to the principle of "here and now" concerning your health and give it first priority.

The principle of "here and now" also applies when maintaining the balance between the three qualities of mind. For example, predominant feelings of jealousy, excessive attachment to someone, or separating from someone you love, brings mental suffering. This state of mind reduces creativity and efficiency, and will darken your mind with grief. However, if you regularly practice *pranayama* (breathing exercises), and meditate, mental pain and negative qualities will gradually perish in the light of sattva. If your mind is dominated by excessive activity, and you lose the ability to look at yourself critically, the darkness in your mind may lead to depression, or other health problems, such as stomach ulcers, piles, and so on.

The following diagnostic methods will help make you aware of the harmony within you—and its relationship to your surroundings.

I have already described about the fundamental constitution (prakriti) in the previous chapter. Before we go on further with the Ayurvedic diagnosis, it is essential to know how to determine your fundamental constitution, for this is the basis for Ayurvedic health care practices.

PRAKRITI—YOUR CONSTITUTION

Most of us are aware that our food preferences, reactions and effects of nutrients and drugs, and our fundamental way of reacting to situations differ, even from siblings. A mother observes the differences between her babies. According to Ayurveda, the fundamental constitution is something that we have from birth. It is the basis of all our physiological and psychological reactions. To maintain good health and mental equilibrium, we have to consider our basic constitution. In each of the seven types of prakriti described earlier (vata, pitta, kapha, vata-pitta, vata-kapha, pitta-kapha, and the equilibrium of all three humors), variations further occur due to the variability in the proportion and ratio of each humor. It is not difficult to see the basic characters described for each humor and to determine in which category you belong. In my classes, students do that fairly easily. The confusion occurs only when—due to a long-term imbalance—there is a vitiation of one or two humors, and it becomes difficult to ascertain one's Ayurvedic identity.

You must remember that the prakriti of a person does not change at a fundamental level. If you are quick to make decisions, have rapid movements, generally dry skin, and feel cold easily, you have a *vata prakriti*. This fundamental nature will not change throughout your life; however, variation in its extent and degree is possible. Due to your vata prakriti, it is essential to give yourself an oil massage regularly, to speak less, to get enough rest, and to cultivate the habit of thinking before doing. Similarly, you should choose your nutrition and the nature of work you do according to your prakriti. If you have vata prakriti, and your work involves a lot of travel, too much speaking, and makes you lead a hectic life, it might lead to vata vitiation. In this particular case, you have to compensate with meditation, sleep, and rest. A person with *kapha prakriti* is able to maintain balance in that kind of job. On the other hand, kapha people will generally not like to take such a job, as they are home loving and do not like to travel too much.

What I want to convey here is that your basic nature does not change drastically; variations occur due to life situations. I once knew a couple where the kapha man was highly intimidated by a vata wife, whose vata was actually out of balance and she was very nervous and stressed. The husband let her do anything she liked, and drowned more and more in his kapha prakriti, thus leading to vitiation (he was overweight, depressed, and so on). After twenty years of this odd marriage, the wife left and the husband had a kind of awakening. He found another companion who was a balanced person and who inspired him to travel and lead an active life. Thus, he was saved from kapha vitiation and its related ailments. The man did not change his prakriti. His slow and stable response to life, and his ability to make decisions slowly remained, and with the help of his new companion he saved himself from vitiation of this humor.

If you are confused about determining your prakriti, try to recall your behavior and physical reactions during childhood. If you were active, mostly running instead of walking, and your parents were always searching for you, your prakriti is vata. Children with kapha prakriti are easier to bring up than others. Relatively quieter in nature, generally satisfied, and slow and steady movements are signs of kapha types. If you recall that your mother was always running after you with a sweater and you wanted to go out without it even on a cold day, or if you were easily angry with your playmates, you are certainly of pitta prakriti.

From the three fundamental characteristics, you can further determine a mixed prakriti if your reactions are wavering between the two. By observing yourself carefully, you can get an idea of the proportion of two dominant humors. The seventh type of prakriti, where all three humors are in balance, is easy to determine, for people of this category are well balanced and more resistant to ailments when compared to others. However, experience shows that in our times, there are very few people of this type.

In normal work situations, people are sensitive and touchy if they are told, for example, about being nervous, or frantic, or slow, and so on. However, if we bring Ayurveda to our work-culture, people accept these criticisms easily and are willing to change. Why? When we comment on people's behavior and working pattern, they regard it as a personal attack and their pride is hurt. On the other hand, if we discuss behavior in the context of prakriti, the comments are no longer personalized and people do not involve their ego, for they realize that they all have a personality type and a particular way of acting and reacting. Besides, in Ayurveda we offer suggestions to change this behavior and working pattern through nutrition, yogic exercises, breathing practices, etc. Thus they don't feel that to change their work pattern or enhance efficiency, they are left alone to struggle only at the mental level.

Many people are interested in astrology and want to know their future. Once a very famous astrologer told me that he believes that astrology is valuable only in the sense that it provides a guide for the future. Astrology can tell us our aptitudes and personality traits. In Indian astrology, people are also told their *prakriti*. It is not our present theme to go into the details of all of this, but I would like to convey that it is impossible to predict the future exactly, whether it is about health or about the political gains of world leaders. The individual's present karma interferes in the prediction of the future. Individual freedom lies in the sense of discretion and intellect (*buddhi*) that we all possess, and which enables us to make decisions about our actions (our *karma*).

We are each born with a particular constitution and its determination should show us the way to keep our mental and physical equilibrium. We can also understand others better when we recognize that there are different types and that each type must follow its path.

DIAGNOSIS AND CARE

It is essential to determine the state of your health at the level of three vital forces—the body humors. I begin with some simple daily observations which do not require any extra time or energy, but just your attention to yourself and to different bodily phenomena.

When you get up in the morning, think about how your sleep was, how your body feels, and how you look after a night's rest. If you feel stiff in the morning, you have to take care of your diminished vata, and if you feel like sleeping more, then your kapha is certainly not functioning properly. If you have a dry mouth, especially upon getting up in the morning, you have diminished vata. Bitter and sweet tastes in the mouth are indicative of pitta and kapha vitiation respectively.

When you go to the bathroom upon waking up, observe carefully your urine and stool. A muddy, thick, dull-colored urine in reduced quantity indicates vata. Yellow and reddish urine is the indication of pitta domination, and foamy urine denotes kapha. A healthy person should have clear urine without any foam.

How are your bowel movements? Does the stool come out easily? Observe your stool carefully. A hard, dark colored stool indicates vata, and liquid, greenish-bluish stool is indicative of pitta domination. A whitish, slimy, and sticky stool indicates kapha. A healthy person's stool should be neither too hard nor too liquid, and should come out easily. It is excellent if you move your bowels twice a day, morning and evening. But it is absolutely essential to evacuate once a day, otherwise ill effects, such as uneasiness and discomfort, are felt.

For good health and longevity, I highly recommend that you drink between 1–$\frac{1}{2}$ to 2 cups (300 to 500 ml) hot water upon getting up in the morning. During the hot season, you may drink water at room temperature. It should be plain water and not an herbal tea or some other drink. Do not lie down or recline after drinking hot water. Move around, do some yoga exercises or other morning activities, such as cleaning your teeth, etc. The early morning hot water cleans your urinary system and intestines. You should consider this practice as important as brushing your teeth or taking a shower. Just as you feel uncomfortable if you don't take a shower if you are used to taking one every day, similarly, if you clean your insides with this simple practice, you will realize the importance of this daily inner cleaning. Besides, this practice brings vata into balance, and it has a tranquilizing effect on the whole body. This costless, non-time-consuming practice is a very precious investment for your later years.

When cleaning your teeth, use a good toothpaste. Some excellent Ayurvedic toothpastes are available. While brushing your teeth, bring your entire concentration to the process; do this activity with indulgence and make sure to clean your teeth in all directions. After having rinsed your mouth, clean your tongue by rubbing a soft toothbrush on it or use a tongue cleaner.[4] Stick out your tongue as far as you can to clean the deeper part. This process will create a sound; it will make your stomach retract a little, and will help clean the lower part of the throat. It is good for those who suffer from chronic bad throats.

Attend to bleeding gums without delay and don't use formaldehyde preparations or other strong chemicals to suppress the bleeding. In Ayurveda, as well as in most ethnic cultures of the world, there are excellent plant preparations that are used for strengthening gums and teeth. The key to good teeth and gums lies in not eating between meals and rinsing your mouth with water after you have eaten something—it may be a meal, a piece of cake, or a small chocolate.

Cleaning your body when taking a shower or bath should not be a mechanical activity. You don't have to spend extra time, you just need to be with yourself during this process—consciously with every part of your body. Use coconut or sesame oil after washing, especially if you suffer from dry skin or live in a dry climate. Skin is vulnerable to vata as it is exposed to air, and you

---

[4]Tongue cleaners can be purchased in health food stores.

should rub your body with oil at least once a week. Wash it with warm water a few hours after applying the oil.

Massage the upper lobes of your ears and your toes with oil during your daily shower. Sniff some mustard oil during your daily washing process. You do this by putting a finger smeared with oil in the nasal passage and then inhaling. This will make you sneeze. Blow your nose strongly after this. It is done to remove any obstruction of mucus in the nasal passage to ensure the smooth intake of air and to rejuvenate your sense of smell.

Give your head a light massage with your fingers while you shampoo your hair. It is recommended to use a light shampoo or a genuine Ayurvedic shampoo. Oil your hair once a week with some herbal hair oil. You can also use sesame, coconut, or olive oil. You may keep the oil in your hair for half a day or overnight, but use an old bed sheet or towel on your pillow so you don't oil up your bed! Oiling your hair regularly prevents hair loss and makes the hair soft and beautiful. Do not shampoo your hair too frequently. Combing your hair rejuvenates the roots, so make sure that you comb your hair as well as brushing it.

The above instructions deal with four senses out of five. For the sense of sight, it is essential to rejuvenate the eyes with some eye drops. Decoctions made from licorice or basilica or chamomile are very good for this purpose. If nothing is available, or if it is too cumbersome to carry for those who travel a lot, use a few drops of your own urine from the first urine in the morning, or use your own saliva. Lotus honey is highly recommended for the eyes and it is marketed by some Ayurvedic concerns. If this is not available, take some other good quality honey. Honey should be used only before going to bed or when you have some time to keep your eyes closed after its use.

It is very important to do some rejuvenating exercises for the eyes. The simplest of them all is the circular movements of the eyeballs. This can be done anywhere during any part of the day, except after traveling or when you are tired. First move the eyeballs up, then down, then sideways to the left and to the right. If your eyes hurt while doing all this, then do this practice slowly for a short time. Gradually, this obstruction will be removed. It is usually caused by a kapha diminishment. The next step is to slowly make circular movements with your eyeballs (fig. 8, page 30).

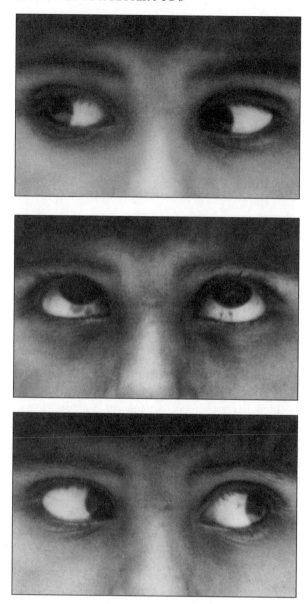

Figure 8. Circular eye movements.

Make sure that your posture is relaxed while doing this exercise. Let your whole body relax.

Concentrating on the reflection of the sun on the water is excellent for the eyes. This may be done from time to time when you are on holiday or happen to be near water. Concentrating on the setting or rising sun is also beneficial in the same way. These exercises are not easy to incorporate into your daily routine, but keep them in mind, and do them whenever there is an opportunity.

REVITALIZING WITH YOGA

To keep your state of health and to make it last until the late years of your life, you need to incorporate some yoga exercise and breathing practices into your daily routine. Many people dispense with this good deed by saying that they do not have time. But people don't avoid brushing their teeth or taking a shower, or eating for several days because of lack of time! These activities are considered absolutely essential and indispensable, whereas yoga exercises or other healthful activities are considered optional. I suggest that you take 10 minutes for yoga and 6 minutes for breathing exercises daily. These should be considered as important and essential as your meals and other necessities of life.

The investment of 16 minutes a day will bring both short and long term gains. The yoga exercises and breathing practices will revitalize your body and its internal organs; they will make you flexible and beautiful. They will enhance longevity and will keep you active, even in your old age. They will also help maintain the balance of the three qualities of the mind by enhancing sattva.

Other modes of physical exercise, such as aerobics, gymnastics, jogging, etc., are based upon the notion that the body is a machine. From the Ayurvedic point of view, these forms of exercise increase vata in the body as they are done mechanically and fast. For some people, they can even prove harmful. Yoga exercises, on the other hand, are based upon the principles of harmonizing mind and body and they help develop self-control, thus leading to peace and harmony. Yoga brings consciousness about your being, thus developing sensitivity toward problems related to health. Various movements done in slow rhythm and with mental concentration help you detect if there are any internal or external physical problems.

I suggest that when you get up in the morning, and before going to bed at night, you take 3 minutes for breathing exercises and enhancing sattva. Then devote 10 minutes every morning to *surya pranama* or prostration to the sun. The details of the 16-minute program are explained along with illustrations in the chapter on yoga.

KEEPING THE SIX-DIMENSIONAL BALANCE

In the previous chapter, I talked about equilibrium at two levels—physical and mental—and have shown how these six aspects are interconnected and interdependent. At this stage, Ayurvedic wisdom may sound very complex as compared to, for example, Chinese wisdom, where balance is sought between two principle forces—yin and yang; or, where the body is turned into a mechanical system and body and mind are treated as separate entities by modern medicine (allopathy). Eventually all six sides of the star (figure 6, page 15) will become clear and you will understand the complexity. However, for easier comprehension, it is essential to understand Ayurvedic wisdom in the context of the cosmos, and without comparing it to other health care systems you already know. This will facilitate the initial learning process.

Greed and a lack of contentment are the two most prominent evils of our times, and they lead to ill health and misery. Consider, for example, food. Wealthy people all over the world eat more than they need and become prey to all kinds of ailments. Greed—needing to own more and more of everything—makes people work excessively and lead hectic and stressful lives. In our work- and money-oriented culture we forget that our stay on this earth is transitory, and that we should try to make it pleasant and peaceful. The real joy of life lies in the feeling of contentment and satisfaction. This is the most important quality to cultivate to begin healthy living. Even if you take complete care of yourself at the physical level, it is not possible to remain healthy if your mind is dominated by greed and dissatisfaction. These two lead to excess of rajas; they cover the light of sattva with tamas. Excessive activity leads to nervousness, sleep disorders, hypertension, stomach ulcers, and several other ailments. Excess of rajas leads to inertia, ultimately giving rise to depression and other mental ailments.

Sattva creates a balance between action and inertia. In the ancient times, religion used to help us cultivate sattva. However, in modern times, the importance and function of "religion" has diminished and it has become merely ritualistic. We need to practice some kind of "world spirituality" that would be acceptable to most people; one that would help us achieve balance and social harmony. Yoga methods can play an important role in this direction.

Anger, excessive attachment, and a lack of control over your senses are other tamasic qualities of mind which lead to health problems. You should not suppress natural urges: hiccup, flatus, vomiting, hunger, thirst, tears, yawning, sleep, sneezing, breathing fast after exertion, the urge to use a toilet—their suppression leads to many problems. However, there are other urges that need to be controlled: the urge of evil ventures relating to thought, speech, and action; and greed, grief, fear, anger, vanity, envy, or excessive attachment (needing to "own").

Basically, the control of suppressible urges comes from your ability to control your thought process. Mind controls mind and this art comes with regular practice and a desire to achieve this aim. Thus, devoting a few minutes every day to some yogic practice leads to control over the activities of one's mind and paves way for a healthy life.

It is easier to cure imbalance at the humoral level than trying to regain mental equilibrium. For example, if someone gets angry and irritated easily because of disturbed pitta, a diet to pacify pitta and some other simple measures will be helpful to regain balance. If someone has fits of terrible anger and loses control, this person will slowly begin to suffer from pitta vitiation and allied ailments. To teach this person to control his or her suppressible urges will require much more time. I give this example to help you understand that in the six-dimensional equilibrium, the importance of harmony in the three qualities of the mind is foremost, and in many ailments, it is the root cause of the problem.

Our modern way of living is highly vata-dominant. Excessive rajas gives rise to the predominance of vata. In technologically advanced societies, most foods are processed and a large quantity of foods are consumed basa (prepared well in advance). Foods grown with chemical fertilizers are also vata-promoting. Dry food, such as bread or biscuits, and pre-pressed fruit juices also affect this humor, leading to its ultimate vitiation. Noisy environments, and the lack of real leisure and peace are some other factors that will impair vata over a certain period of time. It's important to eat fresh food and use vata-reducing herbs and spices. Take enemas regularly to pacify vata and use *ghee* (butter fat) to cook your meals. Try to have a relaxing and peaceful holiday at least once a year rather than taking a vacation full of activities.

The regular use of alcohol and long hours of sitting may disturb pitta. For harmonizing this humor, try to drink alcohol in moderate quantities and never drink on an empty stomach. Ayurveda recommends that you drink good quality wine and beer with food. As for the long hours of sitting, the problem is generally caused by poor posture. Constant physical pressure is put on the thoracic region which is the site of pitta. This problem is discussed in detail in the later part of the book and solutions are suggested.

Jobs that involve closed offices or where dark rooms are required, or if there is a lack of movement, generally give rise to a kapha imbalance. All desk jobs tend to diminish this humor and bring on weight problems. You should learn to balance your work situation with life outside work and nutrition.

However, most of the time people only do something for their health when there are overt symptoms of an ailment. The purpose of this book is to make you aware that it is important to develop a healthy life-style now so that you prevent yourself from falling into a state of non-health. It is a multidimensional effort that involves awareness and affects your whole life. However, after the initial learning phase, you will realize that you have developed an intuitive knowledge, and it is no longer an effort to keep this equilibrium, but a habit.

3

PURIFICATION OF THE BODY—
THE KEY TO HEALTH AND LONGEVITY

M OST PEOPLE ARE very conscious about physical cleanliness and a pleasant appearance, but they completely ignore what is happening inside their bodies. An accumulation of dirt and toxins inside the body obstructs the passage of vital fluids and makes the blood impure. The purification practices of Ayurveda involve cleaning and revitalizing all the internal systems of the body in order to maintain an optimum energy level, strength, and immunity. An accumulation of dirt within the body may lead to sluggish behavior, fatigue, bad dreams, other sleep-related problems, and ultimately to both minor and major ailments.

We eat and drink all sorts of things. We clean our mouths, and what we do not see, we ignore. Imagine if you decide to use only one glass throughout the year, and in it you take water, beer, orange juice, milk, etc., without washing it. You will get sick even at the thought of it. However, it is not an appropriate simile as the body is a living organism, and it has ways of cleaning itself. If we eat something that is absolutely offensive to the body, it will throw it away in the form of diarrhea or vomiting. The inner lining of the digestive tract is made of epithelial cells and they are constantly renewed. Therefore, the body does not need cleaning as often as your drinking-glass but nevertheless, I suggest that you purify your body internally every six months.

Some health pundits argue that internal cleaning is a natural phenomenon and that animals do not undergo such practices. The answer to this is that animals have what I call "instinctive wisdom" as far as health is concerned. They do not use cola drinks, excessive sugar, salt, preserved food with artificial flavors and colors, out-of-season foods, etc. In case of indigestion, they generally fast and let their system be cleaned in a natural way. It may amaze you that animals have tremendous knowledge about natural medicines. Ayurvedic sages in ancient India learned about several medicinal plants by observing animals and their methods of curing themselves. That is why many medicinal plants are named after animals in Sanskrit.

Human babies also react instinctively in many situations to cure themselves. For example, when babies have an upset stomach or suffer from cough, they refuse to take milk. The mothers immediately get worried and force milk on them. Sometimes, they vomit it, thus doing a purification process in a natural way. As the child grows up, this instinctive quality of being in harmony with nature vanishes due to the influence of our society.

When you eat something poisonous, or the food has turned bad, your body reacts in a natural way, and you vomit or have diarrhea. This is the natural cleansing process of the body. But today, most people, due to ignorance, take medication to check diarrhea or vomiting. This is the wrong thing to do according to Ayurveda. You should not create any hindrance in the natural cleansing process of the body.

There are health experts who believe in practices like drinking too much water, absolute fasting for several days, drinking quarts of fresh juices and soups, etc. According to Ayurvedic wisdom, such drastic measures are not good for the body. Complete fasting is forbidden in Ayurveda as it vitiates vata. Besides, this kind of cleansing is not as specific and thorough as Ayurvedic purification practices.

It is easier to comprehend the need for periodic inner cleaning if we try to look at our insides the same way we do the outside. We clean and beautify ourselves outwardly for the purpose of hygiene. We want to look attractive. We clean ourselves with soaps, shampoos, or with other cleansing products, cover ourselves with protective creams, cut and dye our hair, and cut and shape our nails. Just as we look and feel nice after the bath, similarly the body's internal functions are performed with more efficiency and renewed vigor after the purification practices. I have already mentioned that various purification practices are required to cure out of balance humors and the ailments caused by their vitiation. When we purify the body internally every six months, the humors maintain their balance, and the body's vitality and immunity, which is called *ojas* in Ayurveda, is enhanced. The balanced humors and enhanced ojas save us from illness and slow down the aging process. Thus, Ayurvedic inner cleaning practices upgrade the quality of life.

My experience shows that internal purification practices have a tranquilizing effect on the mind. Our modern lifestyle desensitizes us; it distances us from awareness of our body. My experience shows that during the inner cleaning practices, some people have special dreams about old fears or completely forgotten events of their lives. Others are overpowered by a great desire to cry without understanding the specific reasons for it. By cleaning various body parts, we also initiate a process of cleaning the mind.

PANCHAKARMA, THE FIVE PURIFICATION PRACTICES

In classical Ayurveda, there are five kinds of internal purification practices known as panchakarma. *Panch* means "five," and *karma* means "action." They include two kinds of enemas, emesis (or voluntary vomiting), purgation, and nasya. In addition to the actual practice, there are also preparatory practices that are done before doing panchakarma, and these preparatory practices are known as *purvakarma.* They include massage, unction (or fat cure), and fomentation. The purpose of these is to soften the dirt and toxins sticking to the inner parts of the body so that it can come out easily.

During recent years, panchakarma has been popularized in Europe and America by several Ayurvedic institutes. However, this has been done at a very commercial level and people are given the impression that for internal cleaning, they have to visit an expensive Ayurvedic clinic. It is no doubt true that in the case of illness and severe disorders, the individual may be best handled by an experienced physician. However, in case of healthy people, for the routine twice-a-year cleaning, you can and should learn how to do these practices at home. Appropriate training with a good teacher is suggested. Our aim is to train people in panchakarma during a three week, intensive course in our Himalayan center, so that they can do it independently at home every six months.

The inner cleaning practices described here are adapted so that you can use them at home with simple equipment and easily available products. Later in the chapter, I have also outlined a simple program so you can integrate inner cleaning practices with your work schedule. However, it is essential to know that panchakarma forms an important part of Ayurvedic therapeutics and is a vast field of study. The inner purification practices presented here for maintaining health and balance are inspired from the way Ayurveda is practiced in the daily lives of Indian families who still live the Ayurvedic way.

The fifth practice mentioned above is cleaning the nasal passages and the head. This is known as *nasya* (related to nose) because the medications for cleaning the head region are injected through the nasal passage. Since it is not advisable to do this practice without the help of a physician, I have suggested how you can do a head cleaning through various simple methods of inhalation. Alternative methods of yoga are also suggested for this practice as well as for emesis (voluntary vomiting).

The importance of inner cleaning must be understood before you decide to try it. You wash your body every day; you clean it by rubbing it, and using all kinds of cleansing substances. After washing and drying, you may like to nourish your outer skin with some cream to give it a soft look and protect it from the weather (dry, hot, or cold wind, dust, sun, etc.). You know that if you don't do this, your skin will get dirty and rough, and it will age quickly. You apply the same principles to the inside of your body. First of all, by doing internal cleaning regularly, you avoid accumulating toxins inside. By cleaning this way, you avoid unpleasant body odor, bad breath, or unattractive odors coming from other body parts, as well as avoiding skin disorders, such as pimples, acne, etc. If you do not pay attention to the factors causing these problems and only treat these ailments symptomatically, further complications may develop and an ailment may acquire the dimensions of a disease. However, if you clean and nourish your inner parts regularly, you are able to prevent innate disorders (disorders arising out of an imbalance of humors).

Let me give you an example of enemas: if the intestines are cleaned regularly with herbal decoctions, all the dirt sticking on them is washed away. There is a feeling of relief when the toxins and bad smells are thrown out of the body. The inner lining of your digestive tract contains epithelial cells that also have a secretory function. Their secretion keeps the tract wet and slimy to facilitate the movement of the nutrients. The accumulation of toxins hinders the function of these cells, which means that an enema is going to create a new and healthy balance.

Following the non-unctuous enema described above, I would suggest an unctuous (fat) enema. The unctuous enema will nourish the already cleaned inner parts of the intestines and protect them from dirt particles. Besides, your intestines are also the seat of some food absorption and this function is performed with more efficiency. If you never clean your intestines, the dirt that accumulates there for years slowly makes the blood toxic. Besides causing some common skin ailments, the dirty blood diminishes your power to fight against external attacks (and lowers your immunity).

Just as enemas clean and protect the intestines, an emesis (forced vomiting after the intake of fluids) cleans the upper part of the digestive tract (that is, up to your stomach) and your respiratory tract. Purgation cleans the liver and regulates the body fire (pitta). It is extremely important that your nasal passages are clear so that the inflow of life-giving air (prana) goes inside unhindered. Cleaning the energy channels of the head, which is the seat of your nervous system, with medication through the nasal passages, called inhalation or fumigation, rejuvenates your brain and nerves, and keeps you from having an accumulation of kapha in this area. An accumulation of kapha in the head region can lead to headaches, or a weakening of vision, or a loss of the sense of smell, taste, and hearing, sinusitis, and other ailments.

Massage, unction, and fomentation (done prior to the major cleaning practices) loosen inner dirt, relaxes the body and mind, and also revitalizes other major functions. Sweating takes care of the external covering of the body and throws out toxins from the skin. Unction (fat therapy) enhances vitality and luster and makes you efficient and active.

The purification practices of Ayurveda are beneficial for fighting all kinds of pollution. A regular cleaning hinders the process of accumulation and lessens the effect of pollutants, whether they are in food or in the air we breathe.

When vital functions of the inner organs become sluggish due to an accumulation of toxins, it gradually affects your vitality, your capacity to work, your appearance.

PANCHAKARMA TO SAPTAKARMA

Air pollution and food adulteration and preservation require that we really remember to do these inner purifications. I have added to the classical five (two kinds of enemas, emesis, purgation, and head cleaning), two more (blood purification, and cleaning of the urinary tract) purification practices. I discussed this with my Ayurvedic guide and teacher, Professor Priya Vrat Sharma, in February of 1994. He said that Panchakarma should become Saptakarma (the seven actions) from then on. The details of the technical aspects of these inner cleaning practices and preparations follow. It would be best if you could learn these practices from a teacher. This book will get you started.

Purvakarma or the Preparation for Saptakarma

Before the inner purification practices, it is essential to make an appropriate preparation with two basic techniques. One is anointing (unction), the fat or oil cure, and the other is fomentation (sweating treatment). These two treatments bring your body to a relaxed state and soften the inner parts of the body so that the toxins are easily shed during the cleansing practice. To help you understand this, I will compare it to the outside cleaning. Imagine someone who has extremely dry skin that is dirty and dusty and who needs washing. If you wet this kind of skin and start to apply soap to scrub it properly to get it clean, the process might hurt and even peel off some parts of the skin. The best thing to do in this case would be to gently wash the body with water or even with a mixture of milk and water, and then to give it an oil massage. Cleaning the body with soap should be done several hours after the oil massage, when the skin has absorbed the oil properly. Similarly, you need to soften the internal parts of your body with fat and warmth so that they become soft, can withstand the drug decoctions better, and will shed their dirt easily.

Unction (Anointing)

Oil massage: Anointing should be done both externally and internally. Externally, anointing is done with an oil massage. I always recommend that you take special care of the skin to protect it from vata imbalance, which means that you should apply oil after your bath or shower. (The only people who should *not* do this are those who are overweight.) I recommend that you should do an oil saturation of your body once a week (see instructions that follow). About ten days before you wish to begin saptakarma, anoint your body every third day. Preferably, the massage should be done with three different oils. Do the first massage with ghee, the second with sesame oil, and the third with coconut oil. You may also make your own massage oil with a sesame oil base. However, if you do not have time for this venture, heat the sesame oil until some fumes come out of it. Let it cool down and store it for doing the massage. (Heating the oil thins it so the skin can easily absorb it.) Those interested in making their herbal massage oil should use the recipe on page 46.

Always apply warm ghee or oil to your body. For keeping it warm, either keep it in the sun if the weather allows you to do an outdoor massage, or keep your oil container in another container of hot water. Those of you who have spacious houses and spare ground may build an outdoor wood and fiberglass chamber or one with a thin iron sheet. This chamber can also be built in the form of a pyramid. The main purpose for building a chamber is to use it also for fomentation with dry heat on a sunny day.

Anointing the Body with Oil

Put your massage oil or ghee in a bowl or container with a wide opening so you are able to immerse your fingers in it. Make sure that the oil is warm. You may put this container into another bigger container full of hot water so that it stays hot during the massage. Spread an old sheet or towel on the surface where you sit to avoid getting oil stains on anything you value. With the fingers of your right hand, begin to put oil on your left hand and arm (fig. 9a and b, page 43). Massage gently in the beginning and gradually apply more pressure, pressing on all the joints. Massage your whole arm like that, applying a generous quantity of oil. Now massage the right arm with the left hand. Next use both hands to massage your left foot and then gradually come upward massaging the whole leg (fig. 9c). Press all the joints properly and massage strongly on the thighs. Come to the right foot and leg now. After finishing the right leg, massage the front part of your body with both hands (fig. 9d). Apply oil on your shoulders, neck, and face, leaving out the area around the eyes (fig. 9e). Try to massage your back as much as you can. You may exchange the massage with another person if there is a possibility.

When you have finished putting the oil all over your body, begin again from where you started and repeat the whole process.

Some of you with very dry skin might need to repeat this even a third time. The idea is to saturate the body with oil or ghee until it does not absorb anymore. If you have been doing this practice once a week or from time to time, your body will not need a third application.

After finishing the massage, rest for a few minutes and then take a warm and wet towel and wipe off the extra oil from your body before dressing. It is better to keep the oil on for a day, or overnight, or at least for several hours before taking a hot shower.

This practice has a tranquilizing effect and cures diminished vata. It makes the skin soft, stronger and more resistant against injuries. It makes the complexion smooth and shiny. As purvakarma, it is suggested to repeat the oil saturation at least on two different days with a gap of three or four days in between applications.

Head Massage

You should also massage your head with oil at least once during these sessions. The head massage should be done using sesame, coconut, or olive oil. There are also special Ayurvedic hair oils for

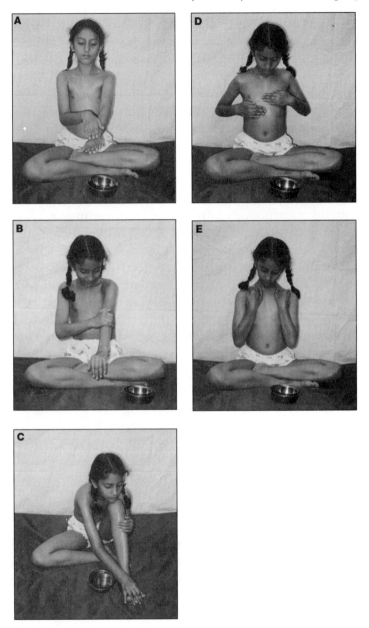

Figure 9. Various steps of self-massage with warm oil for saturating the body.

the care of scalp and hair. Unfortunately, most of the herbs required to prepare this oil are not available outside India. I have provided a simple recipe in case you are able to find the products (see page 47).

Apply the oil with your fingertips on the roots of your hair, and on all parts of the scalp. Massage well so that all the oil is absorbed. You should leave the oil on overnight. Take care to cover your pillow with an old sheet or towel to avoid oil stains.

Fat Intake

Just as an oil massage softens the outer skin, the intake of fat softens the internal parts of the body and helps mobilize accumulated dirt inside. Fat intake cures vata vitiation and that is why some scholars count anointing (unction) as one of the major karma (one of the panchakarma) practices. The intake of fat prior to panchakarma is also important because it gives strength and energy to the body, which you require when undergoing the purification practice. These practices cause temporary weakness and you need to gather your strength before undergoing these purification practices.

Unction taken internally is based upon the principle that if an excessive amount of pure fat is ingested, the body keeps only a certain quantity of the oil or fat and discards the rest. The excess of fat magnetically attracts wastes and toxins and eliminates them from the body. Unction also gives a lustrous complexion.

A simple way to do an inner unction is to drink ghee in hot milk. Take the quantity of ghee according to your digestive power. The recommended dose is up to 6 teaspoons (1 ounce or 25 gm). It is suggested that you should take this for at least three days, beginning with 3 teaspoons, then increasing to 5 and then 6 teaspoons. Add the ghee in about 1 cup (200 ml) very hot milk, stir it well and sweeten to taste. In case you do not or cannot take milk, you may take ghee in hot vegetable or chicken soup. Warm ghee may also be taken as such directly without mixing it in anything.

According to the Ayurvedic texts, ghee pacifies vata and pitta vitiation, enhances vitality and immunity (ojas) and semen. It is cooling and softening, and improves the voice and the complexion.

Before doing this unction, eat a warm and liquid meal that is easy to digest. Do not eat anything cold before or after the administration of the fat. You should not take an inner unction in extremely cold or hot weather. Pregnant women, people having slow or weak digestion, kapha vitiation, depression, or an excess of saliva should not take this unction. Fat people and those who have aversion to food should also not do this.

Fomentation—Sweating Treatment

Sweating alleviates stiffness in muscles and joints and eliminates toxins from the skin, blood, muscles, and fat cells. Fomentation treatment helps remove heaviness from the body and alleviates laziness and drowsiness, thus enhancing the capacity to work.

Fomentation in non-pathological conditions can be done in a very simple manner. It requires heat, either dry or humid, and you are forced to sweat. For general well being, it is advisable to do both kinds of fomentation. After an appropriate amount of sweating when your body relaxes and you get a feeling of well being, you should stop the heat and keep covered with a blanket until all the sweat has dried naturally on your body. You should keep away from drafts during and after fomentation, and you should rest for about an hour afterward. Do not take a hot shower immediately after the fomentation without the prescribed rest.

The Ayurvedic concept of fomentation is different from that of a sauna. In Ayurveda, going from hot to cold is forbidden. This gives a cold shock to the body and disturbs vata.

I have already suggested that you could build a small room in which to take dry fomentation. This room should have walls made at a 45 degree angle facing south and west. If you make this chamber from a metal sheet, paint it black from the inside. This kind of chamber will heat very quickly, even from the winter sun. In countries where there is very little sunshine in winter, you may need artificial heating for this chamber. You can also use a sauna as long as you only partake of the dry heat and you allow yourself to dry naturally. Don't forget to rest afterward.

For wet or humid heat, take a hot bath, preferably with a few drops of eucalyptus and thyme oils in the water. You can also use other etheric oils meant for this purpose. After getting out from

the bath, wrap your wet body in a bathrobe. Get into a prepre-
pared warm bed. You should place a hot water bottle in the bed
beforehand. Cover yourself well and avoid drafts. Get up only
when your sweat has completely dried.

In Ayurveda, the wet fomentation is generally a vapor bath,
which is similar to what we call a "Turkish bath." You may go to a
Turkish bath if one is available, but make sure that you cover
yourself properly after the fomentation, allow yourself to dry naturally, and also rest afterward.

Fomentation makes you thirsty. You should drink something
warm, preferably tea. Do not drink anything cold. You may drink
water at room temperature.

Do not use too much heat, and don't overdo the time you
spend on the process. It should be stopped when you relax, when
the stiffness in the body is gone and you have begun to sweat. An
excess of fomentation or sweating will cause a pitta vitiation,
malaise, thirst, and a burning sensation. Fomentation should be
done about two hours after your last meal. It should not be done
on an empty stomach or immediately after a meal.

After doing an anointing (unction) and fomentation, you
are now prepared for the basic purification practices. You will realize that these preparatory practices produce a feeling of well
being; your body feels more flexible, and your appearance and
complexion improve.

Body Massage Oil

> Sesame oil, 5 cups (1 liter)
> Anise seeds, 2 ounces (50 gm)
> Licorice, 2 ounces (50 gm)
> Chamomile, 2 ounces (50 gm)
> Cress seeds, 2 ounces (50 gm)
> Mustard seed, 2 ounces (50 gm)
> Rose petals (dried), 2 ounces (50 gm)

Powder all the ingredients (except the oil) in a small coffee
grinder or food processor. (You should keep one small grinder
exclusively for herbs and spices.) Before you grind the herbs,
they must be absolutely dry. When they are ground, put 1-$\frac{1}{4}$ cup
(250 ml.) water and the powdered ingredients in a pot and heat

it while stirring. If you feel that the quantity of water is not enough to cook the ingredients, you may add more water. After cooking for 10 to 15 minutes, add the oil and stir well. Let it simmer on a slow fire. Stir from time to time to make sure that the ingredients do not stick to the bottom of the pot. You have to cook it until all the water is evaporated. To test this, hold a spoon or a metal lid on the top of the pot. If there are still traces of water, the humidity will accumulate on the metal surface. While making this oil you have to be very careful and use only low heat otherwise there is a risk that the oil will boil over. Let the oil cool down and then filter it through a cotton cloth. This oil can be stored for several years in a tightly closed glass container.

Head Massage Oil

The basic method for making this oil is the same as above but the products to make it are not available outside India. Brahmi, jatamansi, bhringaraja, and amla should be cooked in same proportion and same manner as above. However, if you have none of these, buy triphala, which is now available at herbal or Ayurvedic shops. It is a mixture of three fruits (amala, harada, and beheda). Combine 10 ounces (250 grams) of triphala to 5 cups (1 liter) of oil and use the same preparation method as above.

SAPTAKARMA—SEVEN PURIFICATION PRACTICES

Enemas

In Ayurvedic texts, it is often mentioned that although an enema only cleans the intestines, it purifies the whole body from head to toe. Enemas cure vata, and since vata is the most vitiated humor of our times, it will cure many ailments caused due to a vata imbalance. Besides, a regular enema will also save us from many ailments of old age by keeping vata balanced, as this period of life is vata-dominant.

When you take an enema, you insert a certain amount of unctuous (oily) or non-unctuous liquid through the anal opening, and keep it there for a while until you have an urge to evac-

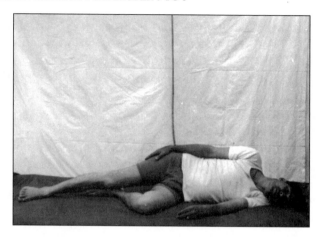

Figure 10. Posture for taking an enema. Before starting the enema, you must hang the apparatus high enough so that the liquid can run into your body easily.

uate. The two kinds of enemas (with and without fat) form two out of seven purification practices.

An enema should not be administered if you are suffering from chest wounds, excessive weakness or fatigue, or after an attack of diarrhea.

To administer an enema, you will need to use enema apparatus. A fairly simple and light enema apparatus can be purchased from medical stores or drugstores nearly everywhere. It consists of a pot (10-cup or 2-liter capacity) and an outlet. A rubber tube measuring 5 feet (1–½ meters) is attached to this outlet, and the end of this tube has a catheter with a small outlet tap to control the flow of the liquid. The enema pot has a small hole in it so you can hang it above you so the liquid will run out properly. You should also have a bench or table to lie down on (fig. 10).

Non-Unctuous Enema

Wash the enema apparatus properly and fill it with warm salty water (½ teaspoon salt for 5 cups or 1 liter of water) or some herbal decoction. Instead of water you could use chamomile, or neem, or a mixture of some bitter drugs that work as a blood purifier and disinfectant. You may use anise or a verbena decoction for pacifying vata and pitta, or a thyme decoction to pacify disturbed kapha. You may also use some other decoction according to your need. A decoction is prepared by boiling the herbs in four times their quantity of water and reducing the liquid to about one fourth by simmering over low heat for a long time. In case the herbs are powdered, you may add only double the quantity of water and reduce it to half.

The normal adult dose for the non-unctuous enema liquid is about 5 cups (1 liter). The temperature of the liquid should be the same as you prefer for a shower. After filling the enema pot and hanging it in an appropriate manner, check the free flow of the liquid by opening the nozzle.

Lie down on your left side with your left leg folded and your right leg straight (fig. 11). Breathe deeply, let yourself completely relax. Make sure that no part of your body is tense and that you are not anxious about what is going to happen. You are simply going to rinse your insides with liquid, just as you wash your physical body every day. Try to repeat a mantra, recite a poem, or use any other method that helps you relax. If you are tense and anxious, you will not be able to hold the liquid inside you, and your enema will be less effective. When you are certain that you are in a completely relaxed state, insert the catheter into your anus and

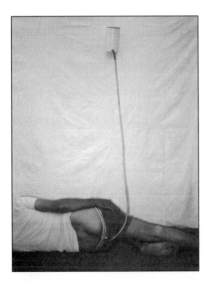

Figure 11. Inserting the enema liquid.

open the tap to introduce the enema liquid. It is advised to smear the anus with some oil beforehand or you should put some oil on the catheter to ensure comfortable insertion.

Some people have a strong urge to evacuate after inserting even a small quantity of the liquid. Try to hold the liquid as long as you can, and if it is not possible, insert the rest of the liquid after evacuation. When all the liquid is inside you, take the catheter out. Stay in a prone position for about 5 minutes, and then take a gentle walk. Keep holding the liquid inside you for at least 10 to 15 minutes.

Normally, you will have to evacuate several times after inserting this enema liquid. Feces, muddy water, and accumulated wind are released from the colon, and you will feel tremendous relief and well being.

After the enema therapy, you should rest. Don't eat for several hours, and then eat a warm light meal. You may eat vegetables, chicken soup, toasted bread, freshly prepared flat bread, wheat porridge, or some other wheat preparation with green and leafy cooked vegetables. You may eat rice with hot soup, but avoid eating rice in the winter. Do not eat salads or other raw vegetables. Avoid sour, hot, or pungent food.

Do not talk too much or too loud after the enema therapy. Do not do any tiring physical exercise or work, and avoid sexual intercourse for a day or two.

Unctuous Enema

The non-unctuous enema should be followed by an unctuous (fat) enema. You can do this several hours later, or the next day. For an unctuous enema, the quantity of the liquid inserted is about 1–$\frac{1}{4}$ cup (250 ml). The simplest recipe for an unctuous enema is a mixture of milk ($\frac{4}{5}$ cup or 160 ml), honey, oil, and ghee (1 ounce or 30 ml each). Warm the ingredients and mix them well. Do not heat above 95°F (35°C) as honey is antagonistic to heat and has a toxic effect if heated. Administer this liquid the same way as before. Let this enema stay inside for several hours if you can. In fact, it will take its own course and will be gradually evacuated. You should rest for several hours after you evacuate. You should eat the same foods as described for the other enema.

Emesis (Voluntary Vomiting)

This practice purifies the upper part of the digestive tract up to the stomach. During the process of voluntary vomiting, pressure is exerted on the upper part of the respiratory tract and this part of the body is also cleaned.

Emesis is done by drinking some warm liquids and forcefully vomiting them out by tickling the deeper part of the throat. This practice cures impaired kapha and is used for the treatment of chronic cough, asthma, and other problems related to the respiratory tract.

Kapha-dominant people can easily vomit, whereas vata- and pitta-dominant people need more effort to throw back the liquid consumed. The number of vomiting impulses during emesis should not be more than eight, as excessive vomiting gives rise to thirst, weakness, mental confusion, vitiation of vata, and the loss of sleep. While vomiting, you should bend at a 45 degree angle and not 90 degrees. That means that you should not bend too much to vomit (fig. 12, page 52). You might need to place a small tub on the wash basin so that you can remain in an appropriate vomiting posture.

The drinks suggested for emesis are soups made from black gram or simply milk. You should drink about 5 cups (1 liter) of one of these and after a short while should vomit it out. One vomit or one impulse is not enough, as all of the liquid does not come out at once. At least three or four times is suggested.

There are many plant drugs suggested in Ayurveda for emetic practices, especially in pathological conditions. For kapha vitiation, you can use licorice. Cook 2 tablespoons powdered licorice in 7-½ cups (1-½ liters) water and reduce the liquid by one third by cooking it on low heat for a long time. Filter it and then add 1 teaspoon rock salt. Mix well before drinking; drink it warm. Keep the liquid inside for about 10 to 15 minutes and then stand in the appropriate posture described earlier. Put your finger in the deeper part of your throat and tickle it a little. Normally, once the process of vomiting is initiated, the other impulses follow. However, if you stop after one or two impulses, you have to excite the impulse once again in a similar manner. Make sure that you do not have more than eight impulses, as excessive vomiting may cause weakness and dehydration.

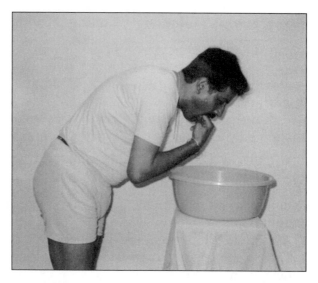

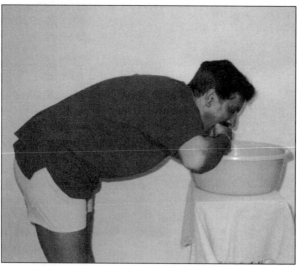

Figure 12. Top: the correct posture for emesis; bottom: the wrong posture for emesis.

Rinse your mouth and throat well and rest after the emetic therapy. Drink some water if you feel thirsty. Eat a warm light meal after about two hours. Specifications for the meal are the same as have been given for enemas earlier in the chapter.

In yoga, there is a practice called *jaladhauti*, which involves drinking warm water, or salted warm water, in the morning and then vomiting it out. I suggest that if you do this once a week, you may not need to do the above-described emetic therapy every six months. With this yogic practice, the process of purification is done gradually and repeatedly, and the thoracic region stays clean and revitalized.

Drink about 2–$\frac{1}{2}$ cups ($\frac{1}{2}$ liter) of warm, salted water ($\frac{1}{4}$ teaspoon of rock salt in 2–$\frac{1}{2}$ cups water), move around a little bit and try to vomit this water by tickling your throat with your fingers. Repeat this two or three times until you feel that the water you drank is gone. This practice will revitalize your stomach, throat, and tracheal region. The taste of the vomited water will indicate the condition of your stomach. If the water is tasteless, your stomach is healthy. A sour or bitter taste indicates that your pitta is vitiated. Foamy or slimy water indicates a kapha vitiation. If you have great difficulty in vomiting this water, that means your vata is imbalanced. This practice cleans the stomach instantaneously, and is highly recommended to keep your stomach in a healthy condition.

When you have indigestion, you should also do jaladhauti, as it provides immediate relief from any stomach ache, headache, or any discomfort of digestive origin.

Do not do emesis if you feel weak or tired.

Purgation (Creating Diarrhea)

Purgation cures disturbed pitta and revitalizes the liver function. It is done by taking some strong purgatives and creating a condition of diarrhea.

You can purchase herbal purgative mixtures from herbal shops and health food stores. There are many specific purgatives available all over the world. In France, there is "Herbasein," in Germany and Austria, I found "Mayr Kur," and in India we take the fruit pulp of amaltas (*Cassia fistula*). I highly recommend the powdered leaves of *Cassia angustifolia*, which is found in many parts of the world. The dose is $\frac{1}{2}$ to $\frac{3}{4}$ teaspoon. The purgatives should be taken at night before going to bed so that they can react on the body while you sleep. The best purgative has a strong reaction but its effect lasts only for one day. Excessive purgation will lead to fatigue, weakness, sleep loss, weight loss, and depression. If you take a purgative that gives rise to only a mild reaction, increase the dose and repeat the next day.

If you feel that you have been over-eating during certain periods of time, you may want to purge yourself to clean and reactivate your system.

PURIFICATION OF THE
HEAD REGION (*NASYAKARMA*)

The nasal passage (*nasya*) is considered the gateway to the head and it opens the way to reach the additional three sense organs located in this area (smell, plus sight, taste, and hearing). To purify the head area, medications are inserted through the nasal passage. This is why we call this practice *nasyakarma*, which means "action with the nasal passage." For revitalizing the four senses and the nervous system, this practice is of vital importance.

An accumulation of kapha in the head region not only affects the sense organs but may also cause gray hair. It relates to sinusitis, and other ailments related to brain and nerves. This purification practice keeps the nasal passage clear. *Prana*, or the life-giving energy which keeps our body and soul together, and keeps us alive, goes through this passage.

Because drugs are inserted through the nasal passage for this purification practice, it is difficult to do on your own. You may need the help of a physician. However, in yoga there are many simple practices for purification that can be used for this purpose. In addition I have discovered some other simple practices that involve the inhalation of medicated vapors or the inhalation of smoke from some special herbs that have proved to be very effective for purification. However, all these practices have a gradual and milder effect compared to the classical method of nasyakarma and therefore need to be done more often.

Inhalation with Medicated Vapors: This is a very simple and effective means of purification of the head region. Oils are readily available for inhalation; they are sold generally to cure the common cold. You may also use some balm, like Tiger Balm or an Ayurvedic balm or other similar product. You can make your own mixture. It is fairly simple to do, and the mixture can be preserved for years. If you want to make your own formula, use the recipe on page 57.

You can buy inhalation apparatus or you can simply work with boiling water in a big ceramic cup. You may wrap a thick sheet of paper around the glass to prevent the loss of vapors (fig. 13). Make sure that you are in a place where there is no draft, and make provisions for spitting or blowing your nose beforehand. Add a few drops of the inhalation oil to your cup of boiling water and begin to inhale the strong vapors. Take a few deep breaths and try to hold the vapors inside you for a few seconds each time. All this may make you cough and you will also need to blow your nose and spit several times. Don't swallow the saliva as it is a part of the purification to spit it out. All this will help clean your excretory glands, clear the nasal passage, and will "melt" the kapha blocking the nearby sinus passages. The word "melt" is a literal translation of what is said in Ayurvedic texts in reference to kapha. This quality of kapha should be understood, like the quality of ghee or coconut oil. These oils melt, given the appropriate temperature, and begin to flow like a liquid. Due to this quality of kapha, kapha ailments get worse during cold weather.

The next step is to take a very deep breath with the vapors and then close your nostrils with the help of your fingers and also

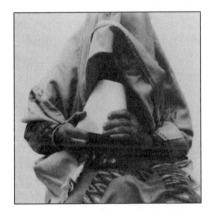

Figure 13. Inhaling the medicated vapors.

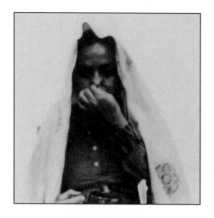 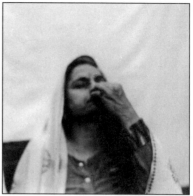

Figure 14: Left: pushing the vapors with force while the nose and the mouth are closed; right: leaning backward with vapors inside while the nose and the mouth are closed.

to close your mouth. Now push the vapors with great force—as if you want to send them everywhere in your head (fig. 14, left). Keep your mouth and nostrils firmly shut while doing this. This practice will make the vapors push toward your ears, sinus passages, and other possible places in the head region. You will feel the effect in the whole head region. Let the vapors out when you cannot hold them any more. Repeat this five to ten times, inhaling normally in between to recapture your breath.

It is quite possible that you do not have enough vapors for the next step. Take a fresh glass of boiling water and add some drops of the inhaling oil once again. This time you are supposed to inhale deeply, close your mouth and nostrils as above, and lean your head backward (fig. 14, right). In the above practice, you opened the passages by pressure, and in this practice, by leaning backward, you are initiating the free flow of the medicated vapors into different parts of the head. Repeat this about five times.

I suggest that this purification practice should be done for five consecutive days during the half yearly purification practices. People who live in polluted areas are advised to do this once a month. To cure certain ailments, such as frequent attacks of cold and cough, hay fever, or asthma, specific instructions are required and they are beyond the scope of this small book on work efficiency.

Fumigation: The other method of head purification is fumigation. This practice is probably difficult to do, especially in the West, but nevertheless I will describe it for your knowledge. It involves burning a mixture of specific herbs. This mixture is put on burning soft coals or burning wood and inhaled through the nasal passage. This could also be done by adding the herbs to self-burning charcoal, which can be purchased in health food stores. The mixture of herbs can also be smoked through the nasal passage with the help of a terra-cotta pipe. The herbs suggested for this purpose are a mixture of equal quantities of licorice, nutmeg, anise, clove, and big cardamom. Mix the powdered herbs together and add 1 teaspoon gradually to create their smoke. While inhaling the smoke, wrap yourself in a towel and lean toward the source of the smoke. Inhale it through the nasal passage, hold your breath and exhale through the mouth.

I have previously described a yogic practice called jalneti,[1] which is very beneficial for cleaning the head area. I strongly recommend it as a regular practice done once a week to save yourself from various infections and from the bad effects of atmospheric pollution.

Inhalation Oil
_____

>   Eucalyptus oil, 2 ounces (50 ml)
>   Anise oil, 1 ounce (25 ml)
>   Citronella oil, 2 ounces (50 ml)
>   Clove oil, 1 ounce (25 ml)
>   Menthol crystals, 2 ounces (50 gm)
>   Camphor, 1 ounce (25 gm)

Mix all the oils* together in a dark colored 16 ounce (400 to 500 ml) glass bottle. Replace the lid and shake well (but not vigorously) so that the camphor and menthol dissolve completely. Do not worry if they do not dissolve immediately, as this preparation takes at least 15 days to ripen. Keep it away from sunlight, prefer-

_____

[1]For details of *jalneti* and of various herbs, refer to my book *Ayurveda: A Way of Life* (York Beach, ME: Samuel Weiser, 1995). The book is also published in German, Spanish, Italian, and Hindi.
*Oils mentioned above should be essential oils.

ably in a cupboard. Shake the mixture gently by simply shaking the bottle for about 3 minutes twice a day for two weeks. Let it lie another week and shake it only 2 or 3 times during this period. Let it lie still for another week and then your inhalation mixture is ready for use.

PURIFICATION OF THE URINARY TRACT

You should always drink water when you get up in the morning (about 2 cups—a large glass). This practice cleans the intestines as well as the urinary system. However, twice a year you should take something strongly diuretic to flush and clean the urinary system completely. Strong diuretic herbal teas are available but most people only use them when they have a bladder, kidney, or urinary tract infection. I suggest that you also use them for purification. In Ayurveda, barley salts are used for this purpose. The dose is $\frac{1}{4}$ teaspoon. You may dissolve the salt in a glass of water and drink it. In any case, whatever you may use for diuresis, drink plenty of liquid so that the purification is thorough and you don't suffer from dehydration. The dose of the substance you use should be determined in such a way that the diuretic effect won't last more than a day. Continue to drink plenty of liquid on the following day.

Blood Purification

In Ayurveda, it is believed that blood gets dirty after a while because of rasa imbalances in nutrition (see chapter 5 for the details of rasas), or by eating foods that don't agree with the nature of the body type. There are many natural products that purify or detoxify the blood. Normally, substances having a bitter taste (rasa) perform this function. Blood purifying preparations also work on the liver and regulate pitta in the body. In fact, your blood is a carrier for pitta substances, but its circulation is the function of vata. The renewal of the blood is a function of kapha. Blood purifiers also cause mild diarrhea as they remove vikriti developed in the body.

However, their function is not only to eliminate waste from the organs of the digestive system. They also clean the blood plasma by removing toxins. People suffering from allergies, skin ailments, or who smell bad need this therapy the most.

Blood purifiers should be taken in very small doses over a period of one week. It is interesting to note that they work differently with different people. Those who have impure blood and who suffer from the above described problems, generally digest the substance for a number of days before it has its purgative effect. People with fewer impurities in their system feel the purging effect almost immediately. Therefore, you may want to prolong the duration of the intake of the blood purifier. All blood purifiers should be taken at night before going to bed.

In Ayurveda, several plants are used to purify the blood, and usually a combination is used to make an effective blood purifier. The two plants having blood purifying effects that are exported from India in large quantities are neem (*Azadirachta indica*) and atees (*Aconitum hetrophylum*). One cannot easily buy an over-the-counter Ayurvedic blood purifier in the West but interested readers may be able to purchase one from an American or British Ayurvedic center.

Bitter teas usually perform this function, and you may decide to take such a tea twice a year for 15 days. For example, you can use a decoction made from wormwood leaves (*Artemisia absinthium*). Other substances easily available are fenugreek, kalonji, garden cress (seeds), coriander, dill, ajwain, basilica, turmeric, and garlic. Besides taking them as a blood purifier, you may also promote their use in your food. Turmeric is an excellent blood purifier and may be taken alone if nothing else is available. In chapter 5, I have given a recipe for the use of curcuma as a medicine (see page 104). You may also make your own blood purifier; see the recipe below.

Blood Purifier

Kalongi	Fenugreek
Cress (seeds)	Wormwood (leaves)
Ajwain	Neem
Basilica (leaves)	Atees

Leave out neem and atees if they are not available. Use the ingredients in equal quantities, let us say $\frac{1}{2}$ ounce (15 gm) each in dried form. Clean them well. Powder them with the help of a coffee grinder. Mix the powder well and store it in a clean and dry container that has a tightly closed lid.

For your twice yearly blood purification, take $\frac{1}{2}$ teaspoon of this powder every evening before going to bed for 15 days. You may put the powder in your mouth and swallow it with a glass of water. The mixture is bitter.

SAPTAKARMA AND TIME

It is normally suggested that these cleaning practices should be done twice a year, after winter and after the monsoons (or summer in America and Europe). That means around the months of September-October and March-April. You may do this in any part of the world, but you should calculate your timing so you do the cleansing practices after the two major seasons that involve extreme changes in temperature or other weather conditions. Some cleaning practices can be used to cure various disorders and may be applied at other times of the year according to your needs, as I have indicated from time to time.

For a regular twice a year cleansing, you do not have to take time off from work and go on a retreat. You may do these practices over a period of few weeks. You may begin with the preparation for saptakarma in the evenings about ten days before you actually want to begin the major cleaning therapy. After you have prepared yourself well with massage, fomentation, and unction, you can do purgation and emesis on the two following weekends. I suggest that if you possibly can incorporate the yoga practice of jaladhauti in your weekly routine, you need not do emetic practice. You may do both kinds of enemas on the following weekend. On the next weekend, keep one day for cleaning the urinary system. Blood purification dose may be combined with other practices, as long as you avoid the days when you do purgation, enemas, and emesis.

You can work in the inhalation practice for cleaning the head in the evenings before going to bed. If you have free time, or if you want to do the cleansing practices over your holidays, keep in mind that you should not do them one after the other. This may cause weakness. Between emesis, purgation, and enemas, you should leave a gap of at least three to five days. You should plan well in advance, but if you feel unwell, tired, or tense, you should postpone your practice. In the beginning, the cleansing practices seem difficult and time consuming. Once you get used to them, they become part of your routine and you begin to realize their invaluable contribution to your life.

4

REJUVENATION
WITH YOGA

YOGA IS ONE of the six principle schools of thought from ancient India. It unfolds the techniques for getting rid of the cycle of birth and death so you can achieve oneness between your individual soul and the Universal soul—which is indestructible and immortal. It is believed that the soul is the real Self of an individual and, unlike the body, it is indestructible. Due to the karma of an individual, the soul undergoes a cycle of life and death. The discipline of yoga teaches us the way to immortality and freedom from this cycle of birth and death.

Yogic practices existed in India from time immemorial but yoga became one of the major schools of thought after Patanjali wrote his treatise in the form of 195 yoga sutras, or aphorisms, around the sixth century B.C. He described the eightfold yogic practices to achieve the aim of the yoga and these are: 1) forebearance; 2) self-discipline; 3) yogic postures, or *asanas*; 4) breathing practices, or *pranayama*; 5) restraint, or indifference of the senses to their objects and their uniformity with the nature of the mind; 6) attention, or *dharana*; 7) contemplation, or *dhyana*; 8) meditation or *samadhi*. The first four steps are at the worldly level, whereas the last four are to overcome existential reality in order to reach the realm of spirituality. To achieve the ultimate aim of yoga, perfection at the physical and mental level is required as both body and mind are the passage to reach the soul. Thus, the first four steps, which are meant to create harmony at the physical and mental level, are preparatory for the next four steps of the eightfold yoga described by Patanjali. For more details of this theme, refer to my book *Patanjali's Yoga and its Practice in Ayurveda.*[1]

---

[1]Vinod Verma, *Patanjali's Yoga and Its Practice in Ayurveda* (Neuhausen am Rheinfall, Switzerland: Urania Verlag, 1998).

YOGA AT WORK

In the present context, my aim is pragmatic, as I wish to help you enhance work proficiency and I use yogic methods to do that. For this purpose I am basically concerned with the third and fourth steps of the eightfold yoga path—the yoga asanas (postures) and pranayama (breathing exercises). In addition to this, I will discuss the general philosophy of yoga from the first and second steps about the fundamental values of life and self-discipline.

Some of the major factors that decelerate your work pace are lethargy, fatigue, listlessness, mental non-acceptance or rejection of something related to work, dislike for the work you are supposed to do, sluggish functions of the internal organs, the mind's inability to concentrate or to "be" in a given moment of time. Various yoga exercises done daily invigorate both body and mind, and enhance your work capacity. You will get a multifold return in terms of your work efficiency after having invested about 16 minutes a day in the practice of yoga. However, I do not claim that yoga alone can cure all the factors that may keep you from doing your job well. The yogic path gives rise to stability of mind, enhances your capacity to concentrate, helps bring balance to the left and right sides of the body and the brain functions, and helps to get rid of lethargy. However, if you are suffering from an acute humor imbalance, you should cure that first with diet and appropriate medication.

I will describe a very easy to follow program that healthy people can use to energize themselves. People who sit at a desk all day long need to move their energy. When they don't, imbalances occur, and these imbalances can be cured by specific yogic exercises. I will also suggest some specific exercises that can be done by a group. If a number of people who work together also do yoga together, they change the vibration of the group, change their ability to concentrate, and generate healthy energy.

Yoga can be used for developing a harmonious relationship with your workplace. Many people suffer from problems related to the atmosphere at work, or they are unhappy because they are not doing what they really want to do. It is very important to learn to use your mental and spiritual strength to make your working environment and the work itself, agreeable and pleasurable. If you are uncomfortable or dissatisfied, your output goes down and you have to use extra energy to perform the most essential duties. This will make you feel exhausted and will drain your strength, which eventually affects your personal life and health.

GENERAL INSTRUCTIONS FOR YOGA PRACTICES

Since yoga involves exercising your internal organs, it should be done on an empty stomach and bladder. The exercises should be done in a peaceful environment and in clean air. If you are doing yoga indoors, open the windows to get fresh air. Wear stretchable or loose clothing. The exercises should be done on a blanket, carpet, or mat spread on the floor.

Before beginning the exercise, bring yourself to a calm and relaxed state. Sit down and let all your body parts relax. Take a few deep breaths by inhaling and exhaling slowly and smoothly.

THE 16-MINUTES-A-DAY PROGRAM

This program is made around the rhythm of the sun. Mother Nature has created days for work and nights for sleep. Every morning, when the universe is lighted once again, you are blessed with another day of life. In Ayurveda, the fire element also symbolizes the intellect. In many languages of the world, knowledge, wisdom, and spiritual experiences are equated to light by using words like brilliant, bright, enlightened, etc. Light gives us power to see with the sense of sight. On a subtle plane, it is this inner light that shows you the way in life. The sun is also a symbol of fame, as it enlightens the universe every morning and its light is everywhere.

This exercise program is divided into three parts. The first 3 minutes are used for breathing exercises to attain stillness of mind immediately upon getting up in the morning. The next 10 minutes are for yogic exercises, called prostration to the sun. The last 3 minutes are devoted again to breathing exercises and to attain inner stillness for getting a rejuvenating sleep. Before I give you the concrete program, I will describe the three aspects that are to be used in this program: 1) technical details of the breathing exercises; 2) yoga postures of prostration to the sun; and 3) yoga practice to experience existence at various levels of consciousness.

Breathing Exercises (Pranayama)

The vital air keeps body and soul together and is called *prana* in Sanskrit. Every time we inhale, we take the cosmic vitality inside our body. Thus, conscious, deep breathing helps enhance the body's vitality. The techniques of breathing exercises or pranayama have four steps:

1) A gradual and smooth inhaling;

2) Holding the vital air inside;

3) A gradual and smooth exhaling;

4) A moment of emptiness without any vital air inside.

Steps 1 and 3 should be done in an equal amount of time, whereas Steps 2 and 4 should take half the time. I do not mean that you should use a watch and time your breathing, but I just want to give you an approximate idea so that you can follow this technique and sense the time intuitively. For example, if you take 10 seconds each for inhaling and exhaling, the time of holding the breath inside and holding the lungs without air should be 5 seconds each.

Within your body there exists a subtle body, with its energy channels everywhere. The purpose of pranayama is to reach these energy channels and revitalize them with prana energy. Thus, inhalation also involves directing the vital air to a particular part of the body. In the present program, I have selected a few exercises to be incorporated in your daily morning and evening routine.

1. The first exercise involves revitalizing the left and right sides of the body separately. Sit down, preferably cross-legged, with your hands on your knees. This posture should be used for all the

breathing exercises. (If you can't do this, sit with your feet on the floor in a straight-backed chair.) Take a few deep breaths in four steps as described above (in 10 seconds, hold 5 seconds, out 10 seconds, empty 5 seconds). Then slowly pick up your right hand and close your right nostril with your thumb (fig. 15, left). Inhale gradually and smoothly from the left nostril by mentally sending the prana energy into all the left parts of your body. As you inhale, let your breath go to the left side of your head, then to the left arm, shoulder, chest, abdomen, and to the left leg all the way to your foot and toes.

When you have finished inhaling, close your left nostril with the help of your ring finger (fig. 15, right). At this time, both your nostrils are closed with your thumb and ring finger. Stay in this position approximately half the time that you took for inhaling the vital air. Lift up the ring finger and exhale gradually the vital air. After doing that, close your left nostril again and stay without air about the same time as you did while you held your breath inside. Then lift the ring finger and inhale in a similar manner as earlier, and repeat the whole practice.

Perform five times on the left side and then five times on the right side. When you are doing the vital breath exercises with the right nostril, remember that it is the left hand you are using to close your nostrils.

2. The second vital breath exercise involves creating a balance between the left and right sides of the body. The basic technique is the same as the first, but this time the breath is inhaled from

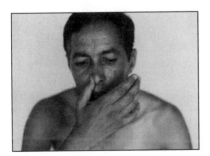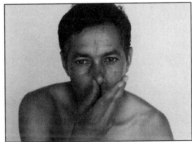

Figure 15. Left: close your right nostril with your thumb; Right: close the left nostril with ring finger.

one side and exhaled from the other. Then the breath is done from the opposite side. First, close your right nostril with your right thumb and inhale gradually using the left nostril. Then close the left nostril with the ring finger and hold the air. Lift the thumb from the right side and exhale slowly and smoothly from the right side. Close the right side again and stay without air. Now lift your thumb and inhale from the right side. In brief, you should inhale from the left side, exhale from the right side, and, for the second phase, you inhale from the right side and exhale from the left side. Do this exercise five times. Remember when you inhale that you are mentally sending vital breath to each part of your body as described in the first exercise.

3. This exercise involves inhaling and exhaling with both nostrils at the same time. Inhale slowly, smoothly, and deeply. Send the vital breath to all parts of your body. When you have finished inhaling, lift up one of your hands and close both nostrils with thumb and ring finger as described above (fig. 15 right, page 67). Hold the breath in and then remove your hand and gradually exhale. Close the nostrils again to hold the body without air. Repeat this exercise 5 times.

4. This exercise is different from the above three. It involves breathing rapidly, as if you have been running for a long time. Breathe in this manner as long as you can with ease. This gives a cool feeling in the head and opens the blocked energy channels in this region. Make sure that you do not do this exercise when tired, pregnant, or after having traveled for a long time. It may lead to giddiness.

This exercise does not form part of the daily program. The reason for describing it here is that it helps you get over the feeling of lethargy and mental fatigue and enhances your capacity to work. It may be done according to your need. I suggest that this exercise be done at work in a group to revitalize the team.

5. After you have achieved mastery of the first three exercises, you should repeat the third exercise except that now you don't close your nostrils while you are holding your breath, or holding the lungs without air. That means that you have developed

enough mastery over various steps of the pranayama practice that you are able to exert self-control. You don't let the air leak when you are holding it inside and you are able to stop the intake of air when you are holding the lungs without air. This exercise is very essential to learn for the practical application of pranayama for protecting yourself against unpleasant atmospheres and infections, and for developing courage. Its practical application will be described later in this chapter.

PROSTRATION TO THE SUN

These exercises should be done after drinking your morning water (see pages 27–28). Prostration to the sun involves twelve different postures which are done one after the other. I suggest that you learn gradually. First learn to do each of the individual postures. Once you are comfortable with them, you can easily do each posture, one after the other.

1. Face the direction of the sun and stand with folded hands and legs slightly apart from each other. Your folded hands should be approximately in the middle of your chest (fig. 16a, page 70). Let yourself completely relax, close your eyes and concentrate on the image of the sun. Your breathing will automatically slow down and you will feel a slight swing in your body.

2. Slowly raise your folded hands upward until your head is between your two arms and bend backward in this position (fig. 16b, page 70). Lean as far back as you comfortably can, making sure that your head is always in between your arms.

3. Straighten your body gradually, unfold your hands and make your arms straight, with both palms facing forward. Bend forward and then downward and touch with your hands the ground on both sides of your feet (fig. 16c, page 70). Make sure that your legs stay straight and knees are not bent. If your body is not flexible enough to touch the ground, do not try to force it. With daily practice, you will be able to achieve this over a period of time.

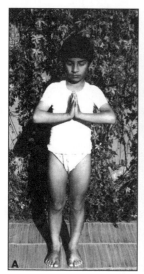
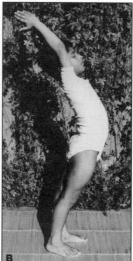
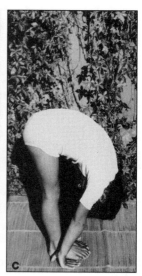

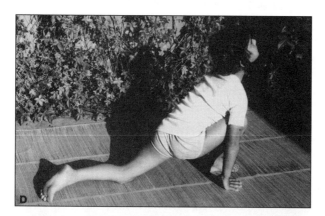

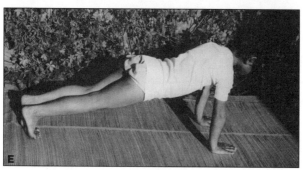

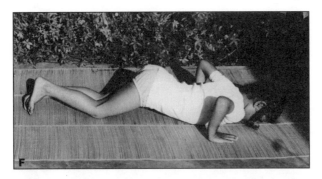

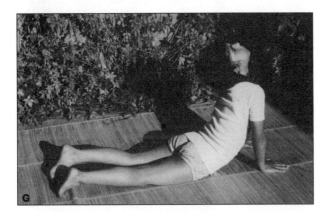

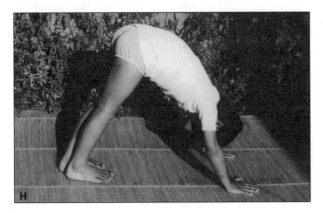

Figure 16. The yoga postures used in "Prostration to the Sun."

4. From the above posture, shift your weight to your hands and your left leg. Stretch the right leg backward so that it rests on the knee and the front part of your foot. In this process, your left leg is folded. Bend your head backward (fig. 16d, page 70).

5. Bring your bent head forward and shift your body weight to both your hands. Stretch back the right leg. Make a straight line with your body by distributing your weight to your hands and toes. Your head should be in line with the rest of your body (fig. 16e, page 70).

6. This position is made by touching the ground with eight parts of your body. In Position 5, you are already touching the ground with four parts of your body—your hands and feet. In addition, now touch the ground with both knees, your chest, and forehead (fig. 16f, page 71). Your stomach and thighs should not touch the ground.

7. Gradually raise your head from the above position by putting your weight on your hands and straightening your arms. Now bend your head backward as far as you comfortably can (fig. 16g, page 71).

8. This position involves making a hillock from your body. Slowly lower your head from the previous position, raise your body in the middle while putting your weight on your hands and feet. Your head should remain between your arms, whereas your feet should be in a flat position with the soles touching the ground (fig. 16h, page 71).

9. Bring the right leg forward, stretch back the left leg, put your weight on your hands and make your arms straight. Bend your head backward. This position is the same as Position 4 (see fig. 16d), except that here the right leg is forward instead of the left leg.

10. This position is the same as Position 3 (fig. 16c). From the previous position, bring your stretched-out leg forward and put this foot parallel to the other foot between your two hands. In

this process, your body will be slightly lifted. Keep your legs straight and do not bend the knees. Bend forward to bring your head close to your knees and lift your back.

11. This position is the same as Position 2 (fig. 16b). Straighten your body from the previous position and raise your arms upward; fold your hands and bend backward as you did in Position 2.

12. This is the last position, and here you come back to Position 1, from where you started (fig. 16a).

CONTROLLING THE MIND

Yoga is not really understood in depth in the West. It has been turned into a sort of slow gymnastics. The so-called meditation is reduced to the level of trying to sit still, cross-legged on the floor, which many find uncomfortable, and during these sessions, there are others who go into a state of half-sleep. The most fundamental aspect of yoga—the control of the activities of your mind—cannot be obtained by attending a daily half hour session. It is a process that has to go on constantly in your mind. It needs no extra time, but it does need constant attention and self-observation. Patanjali describes yoga as "hindering the modifications of the thinking process." The inability to control your thinking process leads to misery and suffering in life. For example, some people are tempted to buy more and more, despite the fact that they cannot afford it. They borrow money and may end up in misery. Not being able to control anger or other emotions may get you into another category of trouble. If you constantly practice control of your thought processes, and gain sufficient self-control by developing inner harmony and stillness, you can experience multiple levels of existence, and can learn to harness your energy in the desired direction. This is only possible by exercising detachment.

When people get into trouble in various life situations they are too attached and too involved with their physical being, or the material things of life. Although in the present context, our

theme is to enhance work efficiency, which also falls into material gain, we want to achieve this in addition to good health and
inner peace. With these motives, it is essential to learn to detach
ourselves so that we can perform our duties with energy and
vigor in a detached state, free from any emotional disturbance
and stress our jobs cause us.

Let me give you an example: Someone in management finds
it difficult to coordinate the work of various people and, from
time to time, literally has to "extract work" from some people
who are relatively inefficient. This process also involves emotional outbursts of irritation, anger, and so on. But the manager
knows that these emotions upset his or her stomach and raise
their blood pressure. This person thinks that the outbursts are effective in the office because they are the only way to get the desired results. The aim here is not to prevent the outbursts, but to
learn—using yogic methods—to keep the emotional outbursts at
a superficial level and not let them pierce deeper in the mind
and disturb the physiological reactions of the body. This means
that his or her reaction is still taking place, but he or she (inner
being), remains uninvolved.

Sometimes, you may require similar emotions to protect
yourself from being exploited on the job. For example, you may
be given an excessive amount of work to do, or you may have to
defend yourself in some other work situation. In life, emotions
are required, as they are the basis of communication. But by exercising detachment, you can protect yourself from the health
hazards that go along with being emotionally caught up in the situation. Anger is useful, but not when it affects digestion.

You can learn detachment by mentally practicing detachment in various life situations. You can calm down the state of
your emotional excitement by chanting the mantra "OM shanti."
Shanti means "peace, harmony" and "stillness." Keep this mantra
in your inner mind, and it will guide you and help you maintain
an inner stillness at every step in your life. For example, in the
next chapter on nutrition, I talk about bringing yourself to a
peaceful mental state and detaching yourself from everything
else in order to devote your energy to life-giving food. Even if you
are with other people, take a deep breath before beginning to eat
your meal, and repeat silently, "OM shanti." Similarly, when you

are in a particular emotional state, remember to repeat the same mantra in your inner mind. You may extend the mantra by adding a word which denotes a particular emotion. For example, for appeasing a state of anger, or the after effect of this emotion, repeat silently in your inner mind, "OM shanti krodha."

You may also chant these mantras aloud if the time and situation permits. "OM shanti lobha" appeases the desire to have more and more. This greed may be for material things, for good food, fame, or any other status or pleasure. Too much attachment gives rise to jealousy, insecurity, a sense of possessiveness, and thus pain. Yogic wisdom says that we came empty-handed to this Earth and we leave without anything, as well. This wisdom gives you mental freedom and inner peace. The mantra for getting over the emotion of excessive attachment to objects or people is "OM shanti moha." Excessive and abnormal sexual desire should be appeased with "OM shanti kama."

By constant effort, you can learn to detach yourself from the negative effect of emotions on your health and you can also get rid of the tamas state of mind, which hinders your mental development and progress.

Speaking too loudly, getting easily excited, or talking too much are other factors that diminish work efficiency and have an ill effect on your health. For the details about the illnesses that are caused by overusing your senses and their cure, see my book *Ayurveda: A Way of Life*.[2] I bring up this subject here, in the context of yoga, to get rid of established habits, through repetitive mental exercises of yoga—mantras and breathing practices. If you speak too loudly, you need to develop a habit of "hearing yourself." By doing so, you will "hear" the jarring effect of your voice and this will inspire you to mend this bad habit. Give yourself time to take a deep breath before you begin to speak. That deep breath is a reminder to preserve your energy for health and longevity rather than wasting it. Think about your physical stamina, vitality, and lifespan the way you think about material wealth. Would you throw your money in the garbage? Would you burn your money or burn the belongings the money can buy? When you speak too

---

[2]Also published by Samuel Weiser. This book has been translated into many languages.

loudly, or too much, or when you listen to extremely loud sounds, you are slowly diminishing your energy resources.

In fact, when you adopt yoga practices as part of your daily routine, you will find that you are gradually developing inner peace and harmony. These two sattvic qualities will bring your mind to work at another level than the rational. At the spiritual level you will develop intuitive wisdom. You will also make fewer mistakes, and you'll make "right choices" because of this inner power. We all have this power lying dormant within us. It is only by developing sattvic qualities that you can evoke this power. Expanding time with sattvic energy will be discussed more in chapter 7.

EXECUTING THE 16-MINUTE PROGRAM

After having discussed various techniques for breathing, prostration to the sun, and controlling the mind, let's see how you can incorporate them into your daily 16-minute program.

The Morning 3 Minutes

Don't begin your day by talking with others (either physically or mentally). Don't jump out of bed and then jump into the shower. By doing so, you lose the substantial amount of energy you gathered during your night's rest. After waking up, slowly sit up and face east. Concentrate your mind on the Sun, the giver of energy and life on our planet. Express your gratitude to this great source of energy for giving you another day of life. Seek blessings for a long and healthy life, and for the well being of all your senses until the end of your life. Then concentrate on your body and on the space it occupies.

Move to a relaxed sitting posture and take 4 to 5 deep breaths. Each time you gently inhale, hold the breath inside for a few seconds, and then gradually exhale. After this, give a slight pause before you inhale the next time. Then repeat the exercise for cleaning the left and right sides (No. 1 breathing exercise). Repeat for each nostril 3 to 5 times. In this tranquil mental state, after having finished these three minutes, think of at least one thing you want to achieve in order to bring sattva into your life. It may be getting rid of a bad habit—bad posture, or a loud voice, or talking too much, or putting undue stress on certain body parts, and so on.

Prostration to the Sun—10 Minutes

These exercises should be done after drinking your morning hot water. If you have learned properly, you will be easily able to repeat the twelve exercises seven times in 10 minutes. If you have more time on weekends or on holidays, I suggest that you take a few more minutes and do these exercises twelve times. But remember, you should not start doing these without any prior preparation. If you are learning yoga for the first time with this book, try to do two or three postures and continue for a week. Then gradually incorporate the whole set into your program. The best way is to learn with an appropriate teacher—one who does not treat yoga as a form of slow gymnastics.

The Evening 3 Minutes

Take 3 minutes before you go to bed; or you can do the following even in bed before you lie down. After taking two or three deep breaths, do the breathing exercises No. 2, 3, and 5 (pages 67–69). Repeat them at least three times each. Make sure that both nostrils are fully open to take prana energy while you sleep. If the nostrils are blocked, or if you feel that there is some obstruction in one of your nostrils, apply some balm or inhale through a mixture of essential oils directly from the bottle (see the recipe in the previous chapter). If the problem still persists, cleanse the head region (nasyakarma) as described in the previous chapter. Remember that during night, your body and mind rejuvenate. An obstruction in one nostril can lead to pain in half the head, weakening the vision in one eye, or it may bring ear problems.

When you finish the breathing exercises, concentrate on the darkness of the night. Show it your gratitude that it exists and that at last you can rest to get over the day's fatigue and hard work. Pray to the night energy to give you a tranquil and profound sleep so you will be fresh and full of energy the next day. If you have a lot of work to do and only a few hours to sleep, ask the night energy to bless you and bestow upon you a deep sleep—so that despite a short sleep you will feel fresh and rejuvenated the next day.

In the process of lying down, repeat the mantra "OM" a few times by taking the prana (or vital energy) to your head.

PRIORITIES FOR THE 16-MINUTE PROGRAM

Try to make this program an essential feature of your existence. It should be as important as bathing or cleaning your teeth. This program helps clean the mind and revitalizes the internal organs. Never ever delete this program entirely from your routine. If you are pressed for time, make it shorter, or do your morning 3 minutes while getting dressed or doing other things. This way, the program remains in your mind. The morning program provides an incentive for the whole day and gives you impetus to work. By concentrating on cosmic energy, you bring the generally rajas-oriented mind to some stillness and expand your "internal vision." Keeping up with this program requires a persistent effort in the beginning but later you will realize it has become an integral part of your life and that its benefits are invaluable.

BALANCING STRESS

Work—the way you do it, the type of work you do, the posture you fall into doing your particular job—may create a physical imbalance. If you don't pay attention, you may wind up with various kinds of work-related aches and pains. These are caused by improper body postures while working—by putting your physical effort and weight on one side more than the other. For example, while sitting or standing, if you put your weight on your left side more than the right, you will gradually create an imbalance. While writing or doing other things, obviously, you put your energy and effort on the working side more (right side mostly, left in case of left-handers). But with conscious effort, and using the relaxation techniques of yoga to balance the body forces while at work, you can save yourself from long term health hazards. Many people suffer from pain in the shoulders, wrists, pectoral muscles, one of the two legs, etc. These are often work-related problems and can be cured with regular yogic exercise. The balancing exercises described below also serve a diagnostic purpose. While turning your body parts in specific directions, you learn where the tension is—the sites of blocked energy.

All over the world, millions suffer from backaches and complications related to their spinal column. These injuries are caused by physical imbalance relating to improper posture while working, or the after-effects of an ailment on one side of the body. In Indian villages, country women do a lot of hard work, but their working postures abide by the nature of their body. They carry pitchers of water on their heads or loads of grass or wood on their backs for great distances, yet their backs remain perfectly healthy throughout their lives. However, urban women in India, who are no longer used to physical labor, are generally complaining of the back pains, particularly spondylitis (inflammation of the vertebrae). Once my friend Rupert Sheldrake, who has lived in India for many years, suggested that I teach Westerners how to carry weight in a balanced way. If I could do this, in a few years we would see people at the Frankfurt, New York, or London airports, carrying weight on their heads rather than dragging their suitcases in one hand and doing damage to themselves. I don't think it is possible to bring this change, but I will make an effort to teach how you can recreate balance after you have done an act leading to imbalance. The six backbone exercises, others for shoulders, and some for reestablishing physical balance are essential. I do not mean to say that you need to do these exercises every day, or that you have to do all of them. You can make your choice according to your working conditions and circumstances. These exercises, done from time to time, will also serve to diagnose the stress points in your body.

The problems of work-related imbalances are enhanced by what I call "working while not working." For example, you use a certain amount of energy to perform a certain specific task, and after the work is finished, or there is a pause, you don't stop the flow of energy you required for that task. For example, you are carrying a heavy bag for a certain period of time, but when you put the bag down, your hand and related muscles of the arm and shoulder remain in that tense work position after you stop carrying the bag. In some cases, the situation is so locked in mentally that the work-related tensions are still there when you go to sleep that night. If you learn to let go when you are done, you not only enhance your work efficiency, but you also save yourself from several long term ailments.

First you need to become aware of these self-created imbalances. Then you can consciously learn to disengage yourself from work as soon as you cease to do that particular piece of work. Observe yourself carefully. Make it a habit to check yourself. Let's say that you are working with a computer. You pause to think about the next idea, or to talk to someone, and so on. Make sure that when you take the break, your fingers do not stay in the tense work posture. Let your hands relax completely. The best technique to use is breathing. Take a breath and send the prana energy to both your hands.

Desk workers, particularly people in management, often suffer from digestive problems. Long hours of sitting strains their site of agni or digestion (solar plexus), and they also have to deal with a range of emotions related to management problems. In addition, people in this category often have "business meals," eating heavy food under stressful conditions. I suggest various yoga techniques to recreate balance. Following are some simple precautions you can take, and some very simple movements you can do while at work so that a particular part of your body is spared extra strain.

1. Always break the long sitting postures by walking a little in between, or at least standing up and stretching.

2. Use a footrest so your feet are lifted up. Make it a habit to stretch back from time to time. You might cross your hands, or put them on your forehead and push back (fig. 17, left). You may stretch your arms upward with both hands joined together to give yourself a good stretch (fig. 17, right). These exercises provide the necessary relaxation for the digestive organs as well as for the hands, arms, shoulders, and back.

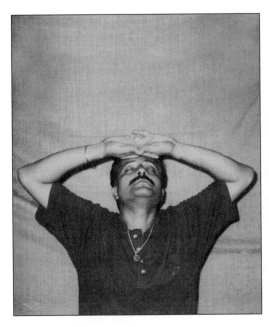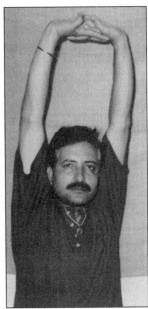

Figure 17. Breaking long working sessions with some simple exercises.

3. Sometimes, you have to sit for a very long time in the same position, as in a meeting. Make sure that your body weight is well-distributed on both sides. In a meeting, when you are paying attention to the speaker on your side, make sure that inadvertently you are not making one of your legs, or arms, or shoulders tense. Many people do so when they are emotionally too involved with a speech, or during a heated argument, or when they feel left out because their ideas are not accepted, and so on. Work circumstances should not have an ill effect on your health directly or indirectly. Remember not to speak too loudly. You can speak strongly without being loud. Use your spiritual power in such circumstances. Before you begin to put forward your ideas, take a deep breath and send the prana energy to your head and to your voice. Breathing deeply will enhance the tone of your voice as well.

During the long sitting sessions in these "very important meetings," make sure that you sit comfortably and not in a tense posture or on the edge of your chair. In between, lean back in your

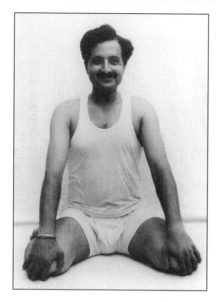 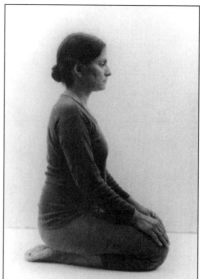

Figure 18. Two versions of the rock posture.

chair and move your abdominal muscles up and down. Remember that this exercise can't be done for two hours after you have eaten.

4. If possible, sit in the rock posture for a minute after lunch. I have shown two versions of rock postures (fig. 18). Those who are unable to make the posture shown in figure 18 left may make the one shown in figure 18 right.[3] This is one posture that you can do after having eaten. I recommend this specially because many sedentary employees suffer from hemorrhoids. This posture is a preventive as well as recommended for those who suffer from this ailment.

5. Don't bend your shoulders while working (fig. 19, page 83). Learn to lean forward in a straight posture (fig. 19, right). The habit of bending your shoulders can give you many shoulder and

---

[3]For the details of rock posture and other yogic exercises for an initiation into yoga for the beginners, see my book *Yoga for Integral Health*, 1991, Hind Pocket Books, New Delhi; German edition, 1988, Windpferd Verlag, Germany.

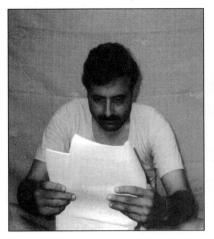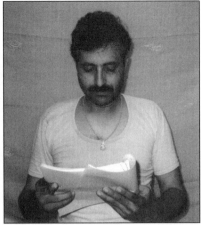

Figure 19. Left: the wrong working posture; note the bent shoulders; Right: the correct working posture.

back problems that may only surface when you get older. In case you have this bad habit, the methods to cure it are described later in this chapter.

6. Make sure the height of your working platform or desk is good for you. Do not work in inconvenient positions where you may have to either stretch your back (or back and legs both if you are standing) too much, or bend over too much. In the former case, you may end up having problems in your lower back and legs, while in the latter case, the middle and upper part of the back and shoulders may get affected. If you work for a while in a situation like this, make sure you regain your equilibrium by doing the six backbone exercises we will discuss now.

YOGA FOR BALANCE

Despite all the precautions you can take, from time to time you will probably fall prey to some physical imbalance and may suffer from feelings of general discomfort, a lack of well being, or from an illness. Therefore, make sure that you learn to diagnose imbalances

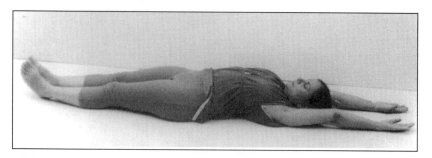

Figure 20. Yoga Position 1.

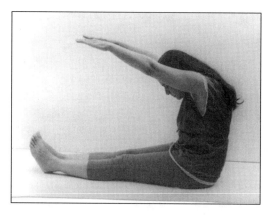

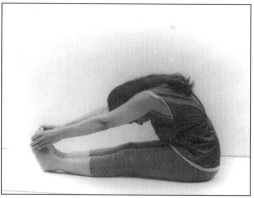

Figure 21. Yoga Position 2. Top: raising yourself up; Bottom: bend forward until your hands touch your feet.

early enough so you are able to cure yourself. I will describe some yogic movements and postures for getting rid of common imbalances caused by working conditions. I also include examples of specific problems, and the exercise combinations that should be followed in order to cure these work-related aches and pains.

1. Position for shoulders and upper part of the back.

Lie down on your back in a relaxed position, with legs slightly apart from each other. Raise your arms in such a way that they are parallel. The palms of your hands should face upward (fig. 20). Hold this posture as long as you are comfortable and gradually increase the time.

If your shoulders are straight, you will have no problem with this posture. If you have forward bent shoulders, you will have difficulty in straightening your arms. Your arms will not touch the floor, and at the level of elbow, they will stay crooked. In fact, this is the posture to cure bent shoulders. If you have bent shoulders, you should do this posture persistently every day to cure it. There are also other techniques to cure bent shoulders, which I will elaborate on later.

2. The forward-stretching posture

This posture is derived from Posture 1. Once you begin to feel comfortable with your arms stretched upward, raise yourself from the lying down position to a sitting position in such a way that, while coming upward, your head stays between your arms (fig. 21). From the sitting position, bend forward in a similar manner until your hands touch your feet, and your head is above your knees or touches your knees. Your knees should not bend (fig. 21, bottom).

Caution: Since you require a very flexible body to do this posture, some of you may have problems with this exercise. One of the major difficulties, which I often encounter with students from the West, is that either their back muscles are not strong enough and they are unable to raise themselves from this supine position to the sitting posture, or they do not know exactly which parts of the body are to be used in this process. While making this effort, your legs are raised upward. Let someone hold your feet firmly to the ground (or floor) and then raise yourself. After doing that a few times your back muscles will be trained, and you will know precisely where to put pressure to raise yourself.

Do not force yourself if you are unable to touch your feet. Go as far as you can each time, and with regular effort, your body will gradually acquire flexibility.

3. The twisted body posture

Make the posture as shown in figure 20 (page 84), and then fold your legs and lift them so that your thighs are almost pressing on your stomach and your feet are lifted in the air. Gradually turn your folded legs on the right side so your right knee touches the ground. In this process, your head and arms should stay in their position (fig. 22). Only the legs should move. Remain in this posture as long as you can. Your breathing will automatically be slower and superficial because of this posture. Move back gradually to come to the original position, give yourself a rest of 2 breaths and turn toward the left side in a similar manner.

This posture will help bring balance to the upper part of the back, your upper arms, and shoulders. If you have been straining on one side more than the other, which is usual with most of us, you will feel the exact place where you are affected. This exercise will help redistribute the energy in this upper region and you will regain your equilibrium.

Caution: In case you feel pain in your shoulders or neck while in this posture, it is a good idea to try some massage therapy, fomentation, with Ayurvedic medicine, or nutrition therapy—which will bring a vata equilibrium in your body.

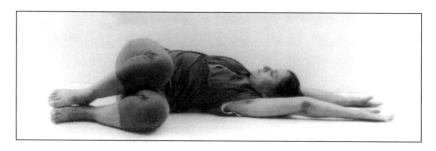

Figure 22. Yoga Position 3. Building on figure 20, touch your right knee to the floor.

4. Six postures for the backbone and back muscles

A large number of people of all ages suffer from various sorts of backaches. These problems can be of diverse origin and it is always wise to undergo a diagnosis. Many of these problems may be originating from bad posture, a curved backbone, or keeping the back muscles tense. The following six exercises help cure minor but nagging back problems, and strengthen the vertebral column as well as the back muscles. They also help to maintain a slim body. *However, you are warned that if you have some grave problem or injury in the back, you should consult a specialist without delay.*

Out of six asanas for the backbone, the first three are done lying on your back, while the other three are done lying on your stomach. These six asanas exercise and revitalize various parts of the backbone and back muscles.

A. Lie down on your back, put your hands slightly apart from your body and join your feet (fig. 23, top). Turn your feet in one

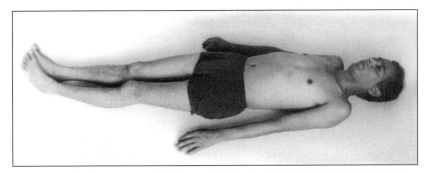

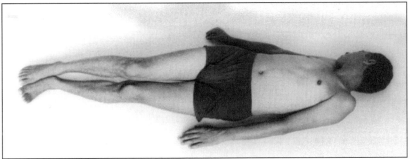

Figure 23. Yoga Position 4A.

direction and your head in the opposite direction while inhaling. Do these movements very slowly and coordinate your intake of air with the movements (fig. 23, bottom, page 87). Once you have reached the farthest end with both your feet and head, let yourself relax and free your body from the efforts of the movement. You will be withholding your breath at this moment. After a few seconds, gradually return to a straight position while exhaling. When you have reached the straight position, give yourself a rest of 3 to 4 breaths. Repeat the same for the opposite direction.

Make sure that your head stretches in the direction of your shoulders and not upward. If you find your neck muscles stiff, do not force yourself to stretch too far out. You will realize that, by doing these exercises regularly, the stiffness will gradually disappear. You will also realize that the upper part of the back is more actively involved. Repeat this exercise four times—more if possible.

B. This asana is similar to Position 4A, except that the position of your feet differs. Instead of placing them parallel, you put one above the other. That means the heel of one foot goes over the toe of the other, as shown in figure 24. You do exactly the same movement as in Yoga Position 4A. Turn your head in one direction and your feet in the other while gradually inhaling and make this asana as shown in figure 24, bottom. When the movement is complete, let yourself relax while holding your breath. The upper part of your foot, which is on the top, should touch the floor in this posture. Come back in a straight position by gradually exhaling and coordinating the movements of the feet and head with it. If you are not flexible enough, and your foot does not touch the ground, do not force yourself. Make an extra effort for about half an inch (1–2 centimeters) each day and your body will acquire flexibility in due course. Pause for a few breaths and then do the posture for the other direction. Repeat four times or more.

This position differs in one way from the previous one as it has two sections. In the second section, repeat the same exercise four times after altering the feet. If your right foot was on the top the first time, repeat the exercise by putting the left foot on top.

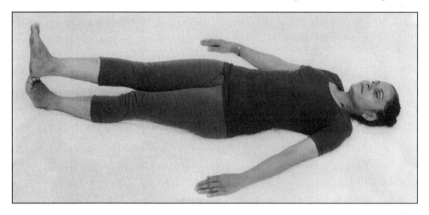

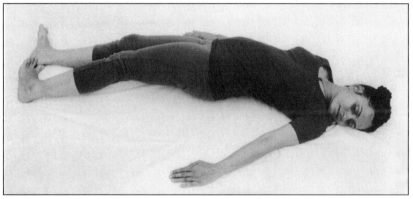

Figure 24. Yoga Position 4B.

While doing this exercise, you will realize that the middle part of your backbone is more actively involved than the rest of the spine.

C. The third posture in this series is made with your legs folded (fig. 25, page 90); the rest of the movements and the position are the same. Turn your folded legs in one direction and your head in the other, while inhaling slowly and smoothly, and coordinate your movements with the breath. The side of your leg should touch the floor as shown in figure 25. However, if your lower back is stiff due to one reason or another, you might have some diffi-

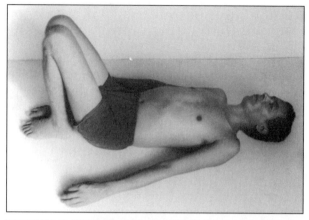

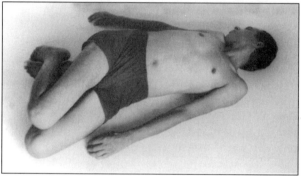

Figure 25. Yoga Position 4C.

culty in touching the floor with your folded legs in these exercises because the lower part of your back is more actively involved than the rest.

These next three positions (4D–F) are essentially the same as the others, but with one major difference—they are done while you lie on your stomach. While lying on your stomach, it is not possible to turn your feet or legs in the opposite direction to your head; thus, you must move in the same direction.

D. Lie down on your stomach with your chin touching the floor and your feet together (fig. 26). Turn both feet and your head in the same direction while inhaling. Both arms should stay at

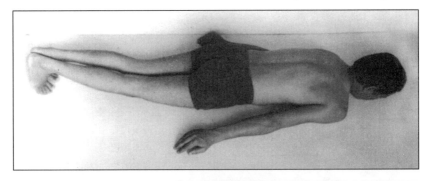

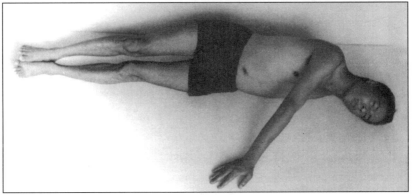

Figure 26. Yoga Position 4D.

their usual place and you will be touching the floor with your cheek while you are in this asana (fig. 26). Maintain the position for a few seconds and hold your breath. Gradually return to the straight position by coordinating your movements with exhalation.

E. The next asana is made by putting your feet one above the other and here, too, like in Yoga Position 4B, you must not forget to alter your foot (fig. 27, page 92).

F. The last of this series involves bending back your legs and then doing the same movements as above until you have made the asana (fig. 28, page 92).

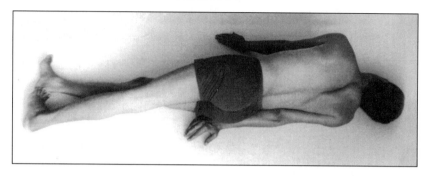

Figure 27. Yoga Position 4E.

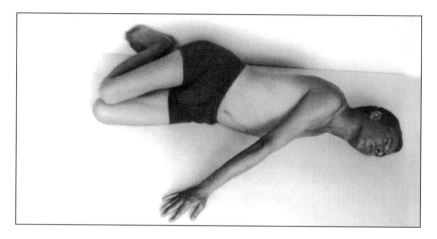

Figure 28. Yoga Position 4F.

Repeat each of these asanas at least four times. You will realize that the last three exercises involve the side musculature of the back.

These backbone positions also help you discover if you have any strain or stiffness in your back and, thus, they are very good diagnostic exercises. This should help you analyze your posture while working. The strain will be caused by putting unequal pressure on your spine, or is due to repeatedly making movements that cause tension. Keep doing these exercises and also

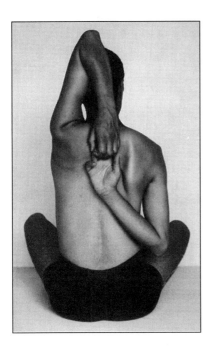

Figure 29. Yoga Position 5.

watch how you react so you can remove the root cause of the problem.

I recommend these exercises to everybody, even for those of you who do not have back problems. For the young and healthy, they are an investment in a healthy back for the later years, and for those over 40, it is already a necessity.

5. The posture for chest, arms, and shoulders.

This posture or asana involves holding both your hands together at your back by bringing them from an upward to a downward position (fig. 29). Sit down cross-legged. Raise one arm up and bend your elbow down in such a way that your bent elbow is behind the middle of your head and your palm is facing your back. Bring your other arm at your back from your waist in such a way that the palm of this hand faces outward. Hook the fingers of both hands with each other as shown in figure 29. Stay in this position for 15–20 seconds when you

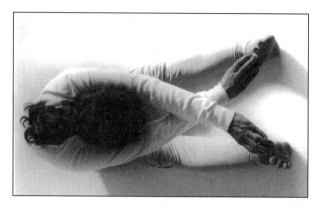

Figure 30. Yoga Position 6.

start, and gradually increase the time. Repeat by alternating the hands.

This position is very beneficial to reestablish balance in your shoulders, arms, and the thoracic region. It strengthens the chest muscles and is particularly recommended for women as it prevents sagging breasts.

You will realize that it is relatively easier to hold the hands together from one side as compared to the other side. This difference denotes an imbalance. Gradually try to balance yourself by repeating these postures. Some of you may not be able to hold your hands together, or there may be a considerable gap between them. Nevertheless, keep doing the posture and each time you do it, make a little effort to diminish the gap between your hands. Gradually, you will be able to strengthen your shoulder and elbow joints and the pectoral muscles will become more flexible.

6. The forward stretch with crossed arms

This posture is essentially the same as the one described in Yoga Position No. 2 (fig. 21, page 84), except that in this asana you place your feet about 2 feet (60 centimeters) apart from each other, and cross your arms while you are lying on your back. Now raise yourself as you would in Yoga Position No. 2. You will obviously touch your right foot with your left hand, and your left foot with your right hand (fig. 30, page 94). *You should only attempt to do this posture after you have perfected Yoga Position No. 2.*

MAINTAINING EQUILIBRIUM

I have described general positions that can be used to re-balance the body when work conditions have helped create back pain. However, some of you may work in special or specific kinds of jobs that also influence posture. I have already talked about the bad effects of sitting at a desk for too many hours. Some of you may stand for long periods of time. Others may be on the phone all day. Another group may work with their hands and feet too much in very specialized jobs. It is beyond the scope of this book to include yoga exercises for all such cases. For example, if you stand for hours on end, you should choose yoga postures that involve raising your legs or bringing your legs into an upward position, or over your head while lying down. You may want to look at my book *Yoga for Integral Health* for exercises for hands, feet, and knees.

People who have to talk too much should do concentration exercises and japa (the silent repetition of a particular mantra) in order to regain their equilibrium. Otherwise, these people will fall prey to various vata ailments. I have noticed that people who talk all day at work like to watch television in the evenings. This, however, creates a further imbalance of vata. These people are using their sense of hearing in excess. The symptoms of vata imbalance are restlessness, sleep disturbance, nervousness, and so on. In fact, watching television is vata-kapha. People whose jobs involve long hours of sitting should also avoid watching television and need to go for a walk in fresh air to maintain balance.

Remember that the effect of the slow imbalance you create may not be apparent so quickly, but gradually you sow the seeds for an illnesss. When a disorder is there, you have to struggle to get healthy again, and sometimes you are unable to regain your health. However, if you are alert and try to restore your state of health, you lessen the chances of major ailments or disorders.

If you have difficulty understanding your particular case and feel that one or several of your troubles may be due to a physical imbalance of one kind or the other, it is best to consult a yoga expert who also has some medical knowledge, a physiotherapist, or a wise general physician.

YOGA ACTIVITIES AT WORK

There are some yoga exercises that can be done at work to invigorate your working capacity and to create an atmosphere of togetherness and friendship. Doing these exercises, which are funny in addition to being beneficial, the sense of togetherness is enhanced, thus giving rise to harmonious working conditions and proficiency. It may not be possible to do all these exercises in certain work situations as two of the exercises are noisy.

1. The laughing exercises

A. This exercise involves laughing very very loud. This is not just about the sound of loud laughing—it's about really laughing in such a way that your whole body participates in this action. You have to build an inner atmosphere of laughing by concentrating your mind so that your laughter is genuine and this process really makes you happy.

This exercise helps relax tension at work; it brings people closer to each other, helps them express themselves freely, and supports better communication. It particularly helps people who are shy, or who have difficulty expressing themselves in a group. It helps get rid of work stress and provides mental refreshment. It takes away the lethargy, makes people active and enhances efficiency. I have great success with this exercise in my seminars, for the exercise enlivens the atmosphere on the one hand, and it enhances the learning capacity of the participants on the other.

B. This exercise is very quiet as it involves laughing without making any sound or lip movement. Your eyes and the rest of your facial expression should show your happiness and inner laughter, but you cannot smile. In the process of making an effort, some people make such funny faces that the whole group ends up laughing. This exercise relieves tension and helps people relax.

2. The lion's cry

This exercise requires that you roar—deeply and loudly from the depths of your throat. Take a deep breath and make this loud sound by forcefully letting go of all the air inside you. It should be a hoarse sound—as the name suggests. The exercise is difficult to explain theoretically and requires a practical demonstration. It releases stress and helps people express themselves freely.

3. Concentrating with rhythm

This exercise involves clapping both hands on the table or on your thighs in a rhythmic manner. Clap once with each hand and count to 4. The next set of clapping should begin from the hand which struck number 4. It sounds quite easy from the description but it isn't in practice. It needs your full concentration, and the moment your attention is diverted, you make a mistake. Gradually enhance the speed of clapping.

This exercise enhances concentration and people have fun doing it. It helps fight stress and breaks tension.

4. Yogic exercises for promoting memory

I am often consulted about problems related to memory and forgetfulness. According to my experience with different people in different parts of the world, I find that many who think they have problems with recall or retention, are actually not paying attention. With a little effort, they can learn to concentrate better and enhance their capabilities. Our mechanized life-style and watching television seem to have influenced a short attention span. In other words, due to excessive rajas and a lack of sattva in our lives, our retention ability is affected.

By following the 16-minute program daily, you will find that your memory improves. To enhance your memory even further, you can use your mind to develop the habit of being always in the present moment. Pay full attention to whatever you are doing at work. Learn to live in the present moment with all your heart and soul. This will improve your general performance as well as enhancing your power of retention.

The present moment is always linked to the past in one way or another, and each moment opens into the future. In your free time, you can do some what I term "recalling exercises." These are done by recalling events or instances of the past in right sequence and with all their details. They could be events in the recent past, or of your childhood, or anything else. Take a few minutes every day to do this exercise. If there is some event that is unclear and vague in your memory, try to recall it again during the next day's recalling session. The "forgotten" event may not come to your mind during the recalling session but at some other time, and it will flash to consciousness. This exercise will help tremendously to promote memory and retention. It also clears up a lot of personal problems so you can move forward with your life unfettered by memories that have been suppressed.

In chapter 8 of this book, I also mention a recipe to strengthen memory. The head purification practice is very helpful in promoting memory. However, all these physiological processes also require the support of your determination and your stillness of mind.

DEVELOPING A HARMONIOUS
RELATIONSHIP WITH YOUR WORK

I meet many people, particularly in the West, who complain of being unhappy at work. They often come to me to discuss quite a different problem, and upon talking to them, it comes out that most of their problems spring out of their work situation. Sometimes it is the boss who is not a pleasant person; at other times other colleagues are the source of unhappiness; or the work itself is not suitable, and so on. Due to the scarcity of new positions, it is not easy to change jobs. In economically developed countries, it is also not easy to start a business of your own. My suggestion to people who feel helpless at the workplace, or who don't like their jobs, is that they should develop inner strength using yoga and learn to protect themselves.

If you find you are not suited to your work, but you have been doing it for years, you can always try to change your attitude about the work. People who don't like their jobs talk about their misery so much that everyone gets tired of listening to them. In this process they lose their friends. If you want to change your life, you should not talk about your work as being unpleasant. By constantly complaining, you are reinforcing your own negative thoughts. It would be better if you could learn to see something positive and good in your work. You could also think of all the people who don't have jobs! The second part of eightfold yoga is self-discipline, and one of the five sections relating to self-discipline is *santosha* or contentment. Try to control your flow of thoughts with the above-described practices and learn to be content. If you do not, you are the ultimate loser, because gradually your state of dissatisfaction will tell upon your health and your outlook on life. You will see everything in negatives instead of positives.

If you have a problem with your boss, or if you feel mistreated on the job, you may want to take a good look at the cause. If your boss is difficult, it may be due to the fact that your boss has problems he or she is not working out. You may be of different types, and therefore you don't relate easily. Look at the types we have discussed. Is your boss being an imbalanced kapha, vata, or pitta type? Are you? If your self-esteem is very low, you need to develop the spiritual side of yourself. You cannot ask your employer to help you develop self-esteem. So far, I have not heard of any employer complaining of employees who did a good job; they usually complain when the employee has "missed the boat." This may be an excellent time to make changes in your outlook so you can begin to like your job. This will have very beneficial effects on your health over the long run.

If you absolutely cannot change you attitude, then detach yourself from your work circumstances. Be like a yogi and tell yourself that you have to work for your survival. You do your duty with a sacred feeling (karma yoga) with full concentration and devotion. Seek spiritual support from pranayama (page 66) and japa (page 154).

If you have a problem related to work, you need to learn to keep *kavacha* (spiritual armor) around you when you enter at the workplace. To do this, you need to practice pranayama regularly. It is explained in Number 5 of the pranayama practices (page 68). Take a deep breath and guide the vital air to the *hridya* or solar plexus. That is where the soul, the cause of our being, re-sides. From this immense source of energy you can make a pro-tective covering around you while you are holding the breath inside. Release the breath gradually afterward. In this process, you will experience a feeling of heat in your body. Tell yourself that with your protective covering, nobody is able to disturb you and you are safe inside your spiritual armor. This is an easy to do visualization technique. You can do it anywhere.

When you leave your workplace, don't drag the problems home with you.[4] Remember that the most important and pre-cious moment of life is NOW—the present time. You should not spoil your present by dragging the unpleasant past into it and worrying about the future. Thus, when you step out of work, pu-rify yourself and leave the problems there. Breathe in using the same technique described above, and take the breath to the solar plexus. Shed your armor there and then. Walk out of the office with a free mind and a sense of contentment.

---

[4]In this context, I mean the problems that are disturbing you should not be dragged home with you. However, there are many times when scientific, intel-lectual, and other creative problems remain in your mind and they need to be solved. My reference is not to these real work problems as they are not trouble-makers.

5

NUTRITION—
NECTAR VERSUS POISON

IN THE MYTHOLOGY of many ancient cultures, nectar (*amrit* in Sanskrit) is delicious: it is strength-promoting and makes you live longer. Opposite to nectar is poison, which tastes bad and may cause suffering and death. The theme of this chapter is nutrition—the food we eat should be nectar and not poison! In Ayurveda, often these two similes are used in relation to the effect of nutrition on our body.

FOOD AND TIME, SPACE,
CONSTITUTION, AND SITUATION

What we eat, how we eat it, and how much we eat—the concept of balanced nutrition—is entirely different in Ayurveda than it is when we talk about modern medicine. Foods are not simply considered good or bad for health, as their effect may vary on each person depending upon the individual constitution, circumstances, consumption, geographic and climatic conditions, age, time, manner of consumption, quality, quantity, and mode of preparation. Depending upon all these various conditions, the same food product may be nourishing, damaging, or medicinal for the body. For example, a glass of cold milk has a medicinal effect for someone suffering from acidity. It has an ill effect on someone who has dominant or diminished kapha. On a hot summer day, a glass of cold milk may relieve the ill effects of heat, while the same glass of milk is damaging if taken on a winter's evening.

Rice is good for pitta dominant persons, during warm weather, and in hot regions. It is not advisable to eat rice at night in the winter. However, when eaten in combination with a pitta-promoting diet, such as potatoes and garlic, it becomes a balanced diet even on a winter's evening! Thus, the concept of balanced nutrition is multidimensional in Ayurveda, as shown in fig. 31 (below). "Any particular condition" in this figure refers to the state of one's general physical condition and circumstances for the consumption of food. For example, when you are doing purification practices, you require a special regimen; during a state of ill-health

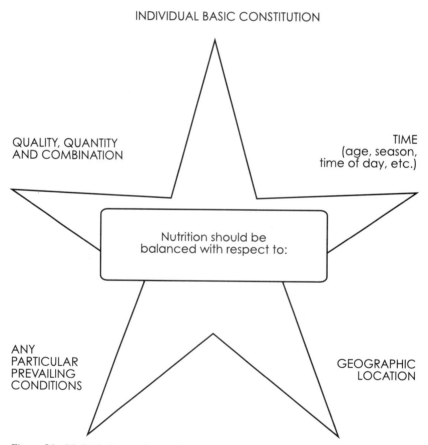

INDIVIDUAL BASIC CONSTITUTION

QUALITY, QUANTITY
AND COMBINATION

TIME
(age, season,
time of day, etc.)

Nutrition should be
balanced with respect to:

ANY
PARTICULAR
PREVAILING
CONDITIONS

GEOGRAPHIC
LOCATION

Figure 31. Multiple factors that are important for nutritional balance.

or some imbalance in body and mind, you need some specific nutrients, and so on. Let us consider another example: someone accidentally falls, or twists some body organ, or has an external injury, such as a cut accompanied by bleeding, etc. In all these cases, vata is activated and an imbalance of this humor may occur. This person requires special food to help the healing process and to maintain the body's balance. A common nutritional cure given in many Indian homes is 1 teaspoon curcuma twice a day (see recipe on page 104). Similarly, for mild indigestion, you should eat more ginger, lemon, ajwain, cumin, and should consume less fat and protein. Or, if you are lethargic, have a desire to sleep excessively, or have a sweet taste in your mouth, you need a kapha balancing diet, such as spicy, astringent, and bitter foods.

Food has other aspects, too. Your mental balance is related to the food you eat. You have already learned that a person's prakriti (fundamental nature) also depicts the personality. External conditions, such as weather or other life circumstances, may change prakriti into vikriti (ill-health), thus bringing also behavioral changes. For example, a person of vata prakriti may become nervous when there are strong winds blowing. However, appropriate nutritional care to counteract the effect of these external changes can influence the emotional state and negative personality and behavioral traits (nervousness, erratic behavior) can be brought under control. Similarly, excessive anger, lethargy, slow reaction time, indecisiveness, etc., can be changed to a certain degree by altering diet and bringing balance to the humors.

Being erratic, nervous, and impatient comes from a vata imbalance. There are many nutritional measures to bring vata into balance. By eating sweet and sour foods, hot, freshly prepared food, avoiding preserved foods in any form, eating regular meals, drinking teas, such as thyme, ginger, basil, etc., and following the other instructions described throughout this book for bringing vata in balance, you can certainly become calm, stable, and even a patient person!

Getting easily irritated and angry is the trait of a pitta imbalance. These traits can be altered by eating foods dominant in bitter and sweet tastes—foods that have less of the fire element—drinking plenty of cold water, cold milk, drinking pitta-reducing teas, such as anise, licorice, etc., and also using all the other techniques described throughout this book for keeping this humor in balance.

Daydreaming, lethargy, slow reactions, and indecisiveness are the traits of a kapha imbalance. These should be handled by eating pungent and astringent foods, and avoiding fats and cold foods. Of course nutritional therapy should be accompanied by the other techniques described throughout this book.

In a contrary situation, if we eat food that brings further imbalance to the humor, we begin to suffer from the ailments relating to that particular humor on the one hand, and a gradual mental imbalance on the other. For example, if a person who has a vata imbalance, or a tendency for that, eats a vata-promoting diet, this may lead to nervousness and sleep disorders. These people are tired at work; they yawn a lot during the day, and their erratic or nervous behavior spoils the work atmosphere. Similarly, when people with an already "hot temperament" eat an excessively pitta-promoting diet, it will enhance anger in them. People with a tendency toward a kapha imbalance may suffer slowed down performance and reaction times if they eat a lot of fatty fried foods, too many grains, or too many sweets.

Thus, we see how the wrong foods can diminish productivity as well as creating a tense atmosphere at work. We can manage our work better, and save ourselves from stress and tension by paying appropriate attention to our diet.

Curcuma Cure

You may swallow curcuma straight with some hot water. However, it has a strong smell and a peculiar taste, and most people don't like it. Traditionally, in Indian homes, we use the following recipe. Fry 1 teaspoon of powdered curcuma with 1 teaspoon ghee for about 30 seconds. Add ½ to 1 cup (100 to 200 ml) milk, depending upon your capacity to take milk. Add some sugar according to taste. Bring to a boil. Drink it hot.

If you do not use milk, or cannot drink milk, you may just eat the fried curcuma with sugar. Soy milk cannot be used to replace cow's milk, as soy has completely different Ayurvedic properties. It is vata-pitta promoting and is heavy to digest. "Cold" in its Ayurvedic nature, the cow's milk, when added to curcuma, makes a balanced preparation.

AYURVEDIC NUTRITION

Before I discuss various concepts of Ayurvedic nutrition in detail, let me explain the logic behind all this. The material reality of the universe includes our physical being, all we consume, and our environment, and is made up of the five basic elements (ether, air, fire, water, earth). Basically, Ayurveda aims to maintain the equilibrium between these five elements despite our constant interaction with the outer world. The five elements, which work as three vital forces in our bodies and perform all physical and mental functions, are constantly affected by time, space, and our nutrition. Thus, our physical five elements are constantly altered by the intake of food.

SIX RASAS FROM FIVE ELEMENTS

Just as the five elements are present in the form of humors in the body and in food, they are also present in the form of the six rasas. The word *rasa* literally means "taste," but in pharmaceutical terms, it means the total effect of that particular taste on the body. The tongue detects the taste of a particular substance and identifies it as sweet, sour, bitter, etc., and the total effect of that particular taste on the body—if we consume it—is called a rasa.

Let me give you an example to facilitate the understanding of rasa. Imagine that there is a small accident at work and someone gets a cut that begins to bleed. You see a red fluid coming out of the wound. Your previous experience and logic tells you that it is blood. That means that your sense of sight has verified that you are seeing a wound and the blood coming out of it. This incident will affect the people who see it differently, depending upon their previous experience and nature. You may be very quick to prepare for first aid, whereas another individual may feel very nervous. There could be another person in the group who cannot witness such a scene, and another may need consolation, or may need to go to the toilet. The sight of a wound, blood, and the suffering individual has an effect on your mind and body. Similarly, when you eat something, your sense of taste specifies the taste of the food. However, that substance with its particular taste, which we consume, has an effect on the body and mind and that is what a rasa is.

Each rasa has an effect on a humor or humors depending upon the elements from which it is derived. Ayurvedic balanced nutrition appropriately combines rasas so that the five elements are in balance. Ayurvedic pharmacology is also based upon the rasa theory. When working with drugs, the aim is not only to supply a substance targeted at the disease, but the drugs should be related in terms of rasas in order to balance the humors. The rasa theory also applies to nutritional therapy when ailments are innate (i.e., due to an imbalance of the humors).

The six rasas are:

sweet, sour, saline,
pungent, bitter, and astringent.

Each rasa combines two basic elements:

Sweet is from earth and water;
Sour is from fire and water;
Saline is from fire and earth;
Pungent is from fire and air;
Bitter is from ether and air;
and Astringent is from earth and air
(see fig. 32, page 107).

Following are some details of each rasa and its effect on the body.

1. Sweet—derived from earth and water: is cold in nature; promotes kapha, but calms down vata and pitta. In this category are not only sugar and honey, but also grains, such as wheat, rice, etc., and many kinds of vegetables and fruits. Some substances are exceptions, for, despite having a sweet rasa, they do not promote kapha. These are honey, candy sugar, wild game, old rice, barley, wheat, and mung beans.

2. Sour—derived from fire and water: is pitta- and kapha-promoting, and brings aggravated vata into balance. Exceptions to

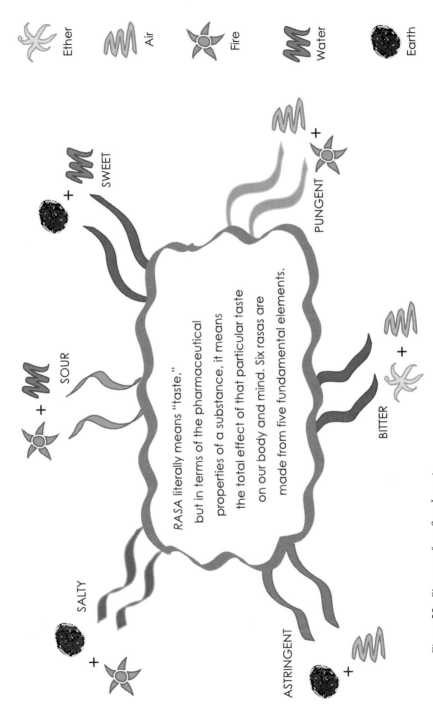

RASA literally means "taste," but in terms of the pharmaceutical properties of a substance, it means the total effect of that particular taste on our body and mind. Six rasas are made from five fundamental elements.

SWEET

SOUR

PUNGENT

BITTER

SALTY

ASTRINGENT

Ether

Air

Fire

Water

Earth

Figure 32. Six rasas from five elements.

Table 1. Relationship of rasas to elements and humors.

RASA	FIVE ELEMENTS	THREE HUMORS		
		VATA	PITTA	KAPHA
1. Sweet	Water + Earth	−	−	+
2. Sour	Fire + Water	−	+	+
3. Saline	Fire + Earth	−	+	+
4. Pungent	Air + Fire	+	+	−
5. Bitter	Ether + Air	+	−	−
6. Astringent	Air + Earth	+	−	−

this are amala[1] and pomegranate, which balance the three humors.

3. Salty (Saline)—derived from water and fire: enhances pitta and kapha, but decreases vata. Rock salt is an exception in this case, as it does not enhance kapha.

4. Pungent—derived from the elements air and fire: increases vata and pitta but decreases kapha. Examples of this rasa are pepper, ginger, garlic, cardamom, bay leaves, basil, etc.

5. Bitter—derived from the elements air and ether: enhances vata but decreases pitta and kapha. Some examples of this rasa are wormwood, neem, and bitter gourd.

6. Astringent—derived from the elements air and earth: enhances vata, but decreases pitta and kapha. Some examples of this rasa are spinach, dates, and jamun (an Asian fruit whose stone is used to control and cure diabetes).

The six rasas, the elements of which they are formed, and their effect on our humors are summed up in Table 1.

---

[1]Amala is a famous Ayurvedic ingredient used in many medicines for both external and internal use. It is a small fruit from a tree that grows in the Himalayan mountains and in North India. Amala contains a lot of iron, and one amala is known to contain as much vitamin C as 2 pounds of oranges. Amala is also a rasayana.

You must remember that natural substances always have more than one rasa and therefore they have several composite pharmaceutical properties. However, in certain substances, a particular rasa is dominant and this determines the principal effect of that substance on your body. Your food is the combination of all the rasas and the skill of Ayurvedic balanced diet lies in making recipes with all the rasas in harmony. All this may seem very complicated from the theoretical point of view, but in practice, after a little training, it is fairly simple to get tuned to Ayurvedic balanced nutrition. A meal should not be dominant in one particular taste, such as extremely sour, pungent, sweet, or salty. Astringent and bitter should be also included in meals, either by using some herbs or by combining certain vegetables. The five elements in the form of the three humors should be balanced with the five elements in the form of the six rasas that we consume (see figure 33).

Various rasas provide us with three vital forces—vata, pitta, and kapha, and thus increase our vitality. There are certain natural products that have several rasas and are called *rasayanas*. A rasayana promotes vitality, immunity, and strength, and provides longevity (figure 34, page 110). Garlic is a rasayana, as it contains

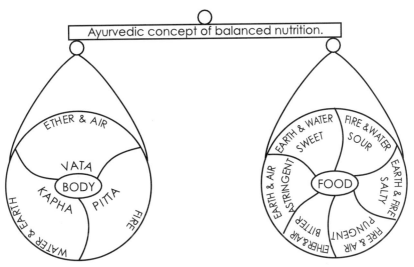

Figure 33. The Ayurvedic concept of balanced nutrition.

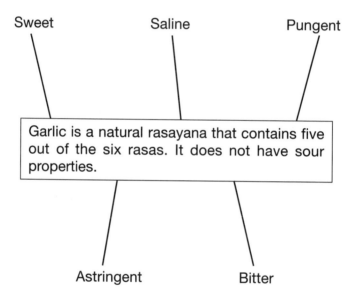

WHAT IS A RASAYANA?

A rasayana is a substance, or a combination of substances, that has several rasas in concentration. Their intake helps balance the body. It invigorates both body and mind by supplying vital dietary elements, or the rasas. The rasayanas also enhance digestion and assimilation. The intake of rasayanas rejuvenates the body by increasing *ojas* (immunity and vitality).

Sweet   Saline   Pungent

Garlic is a natural rasayana that contains five out of the six rasas. It does not have sour properties.

Astringent   Bitter

As a rasayana, garlic should be taken according to one's prakriti: Vata people should have it with ghee, pitta people with crystal sugar and water, and kapha people should eat this with honey.

Figure 34. The definition of a rasayana, along with its most common example from the kitchen—garlic—known as the king of natural substances in some Ayurvedic texts. It is important to eat garlic based on your prakriti so that the humoral balance will not be disturbed.

five out of six rasas. It has all other rasas except sour. Haritaki (*Terminalia chibula*) also contains five rasas excluding only saline. The use of these substances in food preparation is highly recommended.

Whether it is food or rasayana, the intake of natural substances should be done according to your constitution. Lately, the versatile properties of garlic have been extensively advertised. Despite its being a rasayana, it should not be taken in excess (1 to 2 cloves of a medium-sized garlic per day). Vata people should take it with ghee, pitta people with sugar and water, and people with kapha dominant should eat it with honey. You should take it in small quantities, but regularly.

Let's discuss some practical aspects of Ayurvedic nutrition.

FOOD QUALITY AND QUANTITY

Ayurveda emphasizes balance but it does not forbid certain foods, and neither does it propagate that being a vegetarian is essential for good health. Some natural products are by nature balanced (e.g., carrots, turnips, zucchini, ginger, finger millet, etc.) whereas certain others are not balanced, and may disturb the humors if taken in excess (e.g., cabbage, potatoes, cauliflower, etc.). This does not, however, mean that these latter should be avoided. They should be eaten in combination with certain herbs or specific vegetables to make a balanced meal.

There are certain products that react contrary to the nature of the body in terms of properties, combination, processing, place, time, dose, etc., and they are called antagonists. They should be always avoided. See the list of antagonists on page 113.

All foods that are preserved in any way, or that are precooked, are termed as *basa* in Ayurveda and should be strictly avoided. Our modern life-style is vata-oriented with its hectic pace, too many activities, and lack of real leisure, and basa foods add fuel to the fire. Humanity suffers more and more from vata ailments—sleep disorders, aches and pains, constipation, hemorrhoids, nervous disorders, hypertension, etc. Thus, for preventing several ailments, always eat fresh unprocessed foods. Do not drink bottled juices; it is better to drink freshly pressed juices or just water. Bottled juices vitiate vata and give rise to aches and pains in the body. Avoid bread that contains a lot of preservatives; it is better to eat fresh bread or rolls.

The simple practice of preparing a balanced Ayurvedic meal is to enrich it with a variety of ingredients rather than repeatedly eating the same foods over and over again. For example, get into the habit of making mixed vegetables rather than just eating one single vegetable. Use various herbs and spices, such as cumin, ginger, cardamom, basil, coriander, peppermint, etc., regularly in your cooking or to accompany food in one way or the other. The properties of certain commonly used foods and some of the combinations are suggested later in this chapter. For more details of the properties of individual food items and recipes, also consult my previously published book, *Ayurveda for Life.*

You should eat warm meals and avoid cold and dry foods for they enhance vata. Meals should be cooked with some fat as it is necessary for proper digestion and assimilation. "Warm food stimulates the digestive fire, gets digested quickly, has a carminative effect on flatus and reduces mucous."[2]

During recent years, the media has given butter and butter fat (ghee) bad publicity because they supposedly enhance blood cholesterol and thus give rise to disorders, such as hypertension and heart ailments. Ayurveda does not think of equilibrium in terms of eliminating specific foods. Both plant and animal fats are essential for our body, and to cut down on fat all of a sudden enhances vata in the body. You get dry skin, and become nervous and irritable. It is the excessive quantity and wrong combination of foods, accompanied by a lack of physical exercise which cause these ailments over a number of years. They should not be handled by cutting food drastically or by taking strong cholesterol-lowering drugs.

The quantity of food you need depends on your power of digestion, your physical activities, and the quality of the food itself. I will cite a few paragraphs from the Charaka Samhita (6th century B.C.) to illustrate the Ayurvedic views on this theme.

---

[2]Charaka Samhita, Vimanasthanam, I, 24 (1).

ANTAGONISTS IN FOOD

Antagonists are substances, actions, or preparations that react contrary to the nature of the body. The antagonism may be caused by various food combinations, the properties of the food itself, processing, place, time, dose, etc. When antagonistic substances are eaten, actions are done, or one subjects oneself to other forms of antagonism in reference to Ayurvedic instructions, they often produce illness. Sometimes, their effect may come in the form of an immediate malaise, whereas at other times a slow effect may take place. In this latter case, the antagonism may lead to a serious disease that develops over a long period of time. Minor ailments due to food antagonisms give rise to chronic ailments. You should be always selective in making various food combinations. Remember that eating antagonistic food is like giving yourself a slow dose of poison. Following is a list of some antagonists:

1. Milk with watermelon;
2. Milk with fish;
3. Milk with radish;
4. Milk with sour things;
5. Honey with wine;
6. Honey in hot drinks;
7. Hot water after taking honey;
8. Cold food after using ghee or other oily food;
9. Sweet and cold food eaten by someone accustomed to pungent and hot, or vice versa;
10. The use of diet, drug, or behavior adverse to a person's practice;
11. Antagonism in processing, like the use of certain food technology which may render food unsuitable;
12. Antagonism from cooking on bad fuel, uncooked, over-cooked or burned food;
13. Not eating according to seasons, such as eating nuts in summer, cold drinks in winter, etc.;
14. Eating yogurt at night;
15. Drinking something too hot or too cold;
16. Combining hot and cold;
17. Eating too salty, too sharp, too pungent, or too sour substances;
18. Not eating according to geographic location, such as eating rough and sharp in arid zones;
19. Intake of vata-vitiating substances by a person indulging in over-work, sexual intercourse, or physical exercise;
20. Using kapha-vitiating substances by a person indulging in too much sleep and laziness;
21. Not eating according to one's constitution.

The antagonism can be stopped because of the small quantity ingested, your strong digestive power, your young age, or with unction, physical exercise, and your own physical strength. To counteract the effect of antagonists, use cleaning measures, such as emesis and purgation, applied in combination with a light and nourishing diet.

Food or any other thing which is liked but is unwholesome and with unpleasant consequences should not be used out of ignorance and carelessness. One should eat warm, unctuous, in proper quantity, after the previous food is digested, non-antagonistic, in favorable place and in all the favorable accessories . . . and with full concentration.

One who saturates oneself excessively with unctuous, sweet, heavy, slimy substances, new cereals, fresh wine, meat of marshy and aquatic animals, milk and its products, jaggery and flour preparations, and at the same time abstains from physical movements, . . suffers from diseases caused by over-saturation if not counteracted promptly.

One having regular physical exercise, taking food only after the previous meal is digested, eating barley and wheat does not suffer from obesity and is relieved of the disorders caused by over-saturation.[3]

There is one general principle in Ayurveda about the quantity of the food we eat. We should never fill more than two thirds of the stomach with all the liquids and solids we consume. The three humors work to digest food and one third of the stomach should be left available for this process. If this is not done, and the stomach is filled to saturation, the humors push up, causing discomfort and giving rise to several ailments related to digestion.

I am often questioned as to how do we know when two thirds of the stomach is filled. When our hunger is appeased and we feel satisfied and not yet "full," we should stop eating. In the beginning, it might seem difficult, as most of us feel good and happy when the stomach is really "full." However, if, with some self-restraint, we get into the habit of eating less, we will experience a feeling of well-being. People who followed this way told me that, after a while, they got so used to eating less that automatically they could not eat a grain more after the required quantity despite all temptations. Actually, our bodies have an intuitive way of knowing about these things, but this natural wisdom is somehow suppressed with our erroneous way of living.

---

[3]Charaka Samhita, Vimanasthanam, I, 23–24 Sutrasthana, XXIII, 3–5; XXIII, 25.

To have control over the quantity of food you consume, especially when the food is good and in great variety, is very difficult. As it is, overeating, and problems caused due to that, are general complaints from the subjects of my data. I must admit that acquiring complete mastery over the right quantity of food, you need to exercise mental discipline. This comes from self-restraint in general. You can use the various yoga and breathing exercises described in the preceding chapter.

I recommend that you do not take too much liquid with meals, and it is advisable to drink water at least an hour after the meal has been finished. According to Ayurvedic tradition, it is not recommended to take juices or milk with principal meals. Soups are eaten in winter, and in the summer—at midday—a light yogurt drink (lassi) is recommended. However, yogurt foods should not be eaten at night. Ancient Ayurvedic texts suggest good quality old wine, or good beer with food.

Never eat again before the previous meal is digested. According to Ayurveda, this has a poisonous effect on the body. Thus, you should strictly avoid eating even small chocolates or snacks between the three or four meals a day that you are used to eating.

It is better to eat four times a day in smaller quantities than to eat just two big meals. Long intervals between meals and not eating when hungry vitiates vata.

The quantity of your food should be decided according to the nature of the food. According to Ayurveda, heavy to digest and rich foods—when taken in a small quantity—are "light," whereas light foods taken in excess are "heavy." Thus, you may enjoy your favorite fried dishes from time to time, but you need to eat them in small quantities.

Ancient Ayurvedic texts have given certain descriptions of heavy and light foods that can help you determine the quantity in your diet. Pulses, lentils, and some grains are heavier to digest than are green and leafy vegetables. Rice is lighter to digest than wheat, and maize is heavier than wheat.

Each of us knows—from our feelings and experiences—which foods are heavy and make us feel uneasy. You should carefully examine the effect of various food products and avoid those that make you uncomfortable and lethargic. Use a light vegetable oil and ghee (clarified butter) for cooking. Maize, co-conut, olive, or sunflower oils are good. Mustard and peanut oils are heavy. Do not use rapeseed oil and avoid buying mixed vegetable oils as this may contain rapeseed oil or other heavy to digest oils.

FOOD CONSUMPTION

Food should be eaten in a pleasant atmosphere and in a cheerful mental state. Don't eat when you are angry, irritated, or dealing with some other emotion. Do not eat while watching violence or other exciting events on television. Before beginning to eat, bring yourself mentally to the activity and try to acquire a peace-ful mental state. Before beginning, you can say a prayer that will bring you mentally to this activity. Look at your food and say something like this in your mind—"May this food act as nectar in my body and provide me with vitality and energy. May this food give me strength and keep me well. I am grateful to nature for providing me this food."

Sometimes you have to travel on the job, or you eat lunch with coworkers. Try to give yourself a moment to bless your food before you begin to eat.

Appropriate accessories and a comfortable place to eat add to the taste of your food and its positive effect on you. Don't gulp your food or eat while standing. Food should be chewed properly and should be eaten neither too slowly nor too fast. Both these actions enhance vata.

AYURVEDIC FOODS

Many people confuse Ayurvedic food with Indian food. Indian food is not "Ayurvedic cooking." There are many books available with only Indian recipes, titled Ayurvedic cooking, but all Indian cooking is not Ayurvedic cooking and Ayurvedic cooking does not have to be Indian! Ayurveda, as a science of life, describes the concept of balanced nutrition, but this balance, as you must have realized by now, is quite complicated. It is what we eat in relation to who we are, and where we are, and how we eat, and so on. If we begin to eat Indian recipes in a cold American or European climate, it may not be a very good idea. Therefore, I will give you some recipes so you can learn the basic ideas and will be able to beneficially use them in your way of cooking.

A balanced and health-promoting diet keeps the humors in balance and enhances ojas (vitality and immunity). The concept of balance may vary if you are living in the mountains or on the seashore. If you move geographically, make sure you change your diet accordingly. Do not insist on eating the fruits and vegetables that you are used to eating. How do the local people live and eat? Try to feel the effect of the new place on yourself and look at that with reference to Ayurvedic wisdom.

Many people in the West, and equally some big city dwellers in India now, do not relate nutrition to time. They eat nuts during the summer months, eat ice cream in the winter, yogurt when they have a fever, eat the same food in youth as in old age, and so on. Odd combinations of foods, such as hot tea or coffee and yogurt, ice cream and beer, etc., which are antagonists, are also consumed. I have tried to point out the major things that cause imbalance and gradually make us sick. Keep in mind the foods that have antagonistic effects for they can make you sick. Avoid them.

The food you cook should taste good in addition to being balanced and rejuvenating. Ayurveda does not recommend health care through suffering, as the lack of pleasure in life will also give rise to disease. That is why, in Ayurveda, special attention has been paid to the culinary arts as well as to sexual fulfillment.

The tradition of Ayurvedic cooking is assimilated in many Indian homes and my idea is that Ayurvedic cooking should be taught in a simple way, as it is done daily in these homes. It should not be taught using ancient Ayurvedic texts as if the reader has to pass an exam. I have explained the technical aspects in simple terms, and I will try to keep this section very practical so that you can really cook the Ayurvedic way rather than getting entangled with all the complicated details.

Foods are divided into hot and cold rather than according to the three humors. Hot enhances pitta, cold enhances kapha and vata. Obviously, summer and winter foods are predominant in cold and hot things respectively. If some vegetable (or meat) is hot in its properties, its preparation for summer requires the addition of particular herbs and spices that are "cold." Urad beans (for availability and other details, see the list of products later in the chapter) are very hot in their properties and in South India, many preparations are made with their flour—along with rice flour, which is cold in nature. Similarly, foods that are cold in nature should be balanced with foods or spices that are hot. One does not have to mix the balancing products in the same recipe; it could be in another form during the meal. For example, if you have rice as a main dish during a winter evening, you could also eat a tomato salad with garlic in the same meal.

Another aspect of Ayurvedic nutrition deals with balance. When you have heavy-to-digest foods, you add those herbs and spices—or make combinations with such things—which promote digestion. For example, fried things are heavy to digest and it is recommended that they be avoided. But when you eat them, you should add ajwain, cumin, kalonji, or ginger (see page 124 for details) depending upon the recipe. Foods that are heavy to digest should be eaten in smaller quantities.

Let me talk some more about the hot and cold nature of foods that are commonly used all over the world. In case you want to find out about products which are not mentioned here, try to apply the fundamental wisdom of rasas. Observe carefully the tastes your tongue feels for that particular substance, look at the rasa table and figure out what could be its humoral effect. Its hot or cold nature will be determined by the dominant taste and subsequently the elements from which this taste originates.

CLASSIFICATION OF MAJOR FOODS

Table 2 classifies food items into three categories: cold, hot, and balanced. In the category of cold foods, I have specifically marked "vata" in parentheses when the foods enhance this humor in particular. These should be balanced with the addition of spice mixtures 2 or 3 (given at the end of the chapter),

Table 2. Food classifications.

FOODS COLD IN NATURE
Grains: Wheat, rice, maize (promotes vata), barley (increases vata), common millet and Italian millet (promotes vata), masoor beans (promotes vata), young green peas, ripe green peas (strongly vata-promoting), chick peas
Vegetables: Spinach, cabbage and Brussels sprouts (vata), okra, green beans, bitter gourd, endives, fennel, aubergine, onion, celery, cucumber, beetroot
Fruits: Apples (sweet), bananas, pears, apricots, guava, musk melon, watermelon, figs
Dairy products: Milk, ghee
Meat: Frog, seafood, sea fish, mutton
Herbs and spices: Cloves, coriander, anise, licorice
Others: Sugar
FOODS HOT IN NATURE
Grains: Urad beans, soya beans
Vegetables: Cress salad, potatoes, cauliflower, tomatoes
Fruits: Oranges, grapefruit, lemon, grapes (which are not absolutely sweet), peaches, plums, kiwi (specifically the black seeds in kiwi), nuts (almonds, peanuts, hazelnuts and others)
Dairy products: Yogurt, processed cheese
Meats: Pork, horse, beef, freshwater fish
Herbs and spices: Greater cardamom, cumin, cinnamon, black pepper, fenugreek, kalonji, garlic, basil, dill seeds, ajwain, mustard seeds
Others: Honey, vegetable oils, eggs (hen, fish)
FOODS TO BRING HUMORAL EQUILIBRIUM
Grains: Finger millet, mung beans, germinated (sprouts) chick peas
Vegetables: Carrots, small radishes (not overripe), turnips, zucchini, pumpkin (just ripened)
Fruits: Sweet mangoes, papaya, pomegranate, grapes (sweet)
Meats: Deer, goat, chicken
Herbs and spices: Small cardamom, ginger, curcuma

garlic, dill seeds, and/or fenugreek. The choice of what you use as spice for pacifying the vata effect depends upon what you are cooking.

RECIPES

Here are some concrete suggestions so that you can directly use them in your everyday cooking. Before we start with the recipes, I will also give some general instructions for using Ayurvedic wisdom in your everyday food and cooking.

1. Whenever you prepare something with flour, try to use some spices that promote digestion. In salty preparations, you may use ajwain, cumin, or kalonji. In sweet preparations, you may use some small cardamom, anise, or cinnamon. Ajwain can also be used in sweet preparations. Ginger can be used in both sweet and salty dishes.

2. Try to eat deep fried foods as seldom as possible. If you are fond of fried foods, orient yourself toward cooking which is delicious even without frying. In any case, whenever you make fried food, do add ajwain in your batter or dough.

3. Make sure that you do not eat the same things over and over. Try to eat a variety. Cook mixed vegetables and grains.

4. Always remember that an excess of anything is bad and try to adopt a middle way. You can drink a moderate quantity of wine or beer. If you are a meat eater, try not to eat too much meat. Also use only moderate quantities of sugar. You should include grains, vegetables, and fruits in your meals. Some people tend to go to extremes with some eating habits. People are given a lot of erroneous information—many books on nutrition are written about personal experience. For example, someone who cured himself or herself from a serious ailment by eating only fruits wants others to benefit from this and pens his or her story. This information may be true but cannot be made into a universal

rule. It is not scientific information, it is merely a case study. Applied to somebody who has a different humoral balance may cause harm.

I will give you a good example to illustrate my statement. Recently, I had a visit from a friend from Switzerland. It was April—hot and dry in the Delhi area, with temperatures around 35° C. This friend is totally convinced that fruits are the healthiest things to eat, that they can prevent and cure even cancer; and he has many fantastic stories to tell in this direction. This person has a pitta prakriti and his pitta is in vikriti very often. Eating a huge amount of fruit in a hot climate, with his pitta vitiation, he made himself really sick. He was angry, irritated, feeling excessive heat in his body, and so on. When his body could not stand all this, it did a natural cleansing process, and to get rid of the excess of pitta, he had a bad case of diarrhea. In this kind of heat, the body needs grains or other solid nutrients that help hold water. Rice, with some cooked vegetables (zucchini, carrots, turnips, etc.), along with some ghee, can be very beneficial to restore the state of health from such a situation.

5. An appropriate use of herbs and spices not only makes food delicious, it also keeps the humors in balance and enhances ojas (immunity and vitality). This latter can save us from many small but nagging ailments. For specific rejuvenating effects, and for curing minor ailments with various spices from the kitchen, see the last chapter of this book. I use herbs and spices in the following recipes. Use them carefully as the spices should balance food preparation. If you make mistakes with the quantity, quality, and the type of the spices used, you can make yourself sick. For example, too much pepper can cause heartburn, excessive use of garlic at the wrong time can give rise to restlessness, thirst, and a dry throat.

Breakfast

When I tell people to eat freshly prepared warm meals, they are at a loss, especially for breakfast. Bread is a "basa" food and too much intake of yeast should be avoided anyway. Let's look for other ways and forms of consuming wheat which are healthier.

However, if you wish to eat a classical breakfast with bread, butter, jam, etc., along with tea or coffee, I suggest that 1) you should toast your bread or eat freshly made bread, such as rolls; 2) don't use salty butter, as the bread already contains salt; 3) if you eat jams, try to prepare them with ginger, also avoid very sour jams; and 4) drink rejuvenating tea as described in the last chapter of this book; black coffee or tea without milk should be avoided.

Wheat Porridge

The best wheat porridge can be prepared from wheat that is slightly sprouted. You can sprout wheat for 24 hours, dry it, and then grind it and keep it for making porridge. Take 1 pound 1-½ ounces of wheat. Clean and wash it well and leave it soaked in very little water, only enough to keep it wet. Leave it like this for about 24 hours or longer if the climate is cold. The wheat just begins to sprout. This state of sprouting is considered the healthiest in Ayurveda. Drain the water and spread the wheat on cotton or linen napkins. It will take several days until it is absolutely dry.

You can use a small coffee grinder to grind this wheat a little if you do not have a bigger grinder. Do not over-grind and make it into small granules or flour. Roughly speaking, keep in mind a size that is about ¼ of a wheat grain. You can store this ground wheat in a clean and dry jar.

For breakfast for one person, fry 2–3 tablespoons of this wheat in 1 teaspoon ghee, until it is slightly brown. Add 1 cup (200 ml) water and let it cook. Add three crushed small cardamoms. Stir from time to time and let it cook for 10 minutes on a low fire. Add about ¾ cup (150 ml) of milk, and sugar to taste, and cook again for 3–4 minutes. You may also add some dry fruits, such as raisins, dates, coconut, or almonds if you wish to have an enriched breakfast. For a very simple breakfast, or for those who do not like to drink milk, you may leave out milk. You may add the dry fruits as mentioned above. You can also leave out the ghee in case you are overweight.

Options: You may make the same recipe with semolina or with grated carrots. To make carrots, take 4 medium-sized carrots, cook them covered, and if at all, add a little sugar. Do not add water, add ¾ cup milk. Cook for 3–4 minutes as you would the wheat. This is a very energy-giving breakfast and I recommend it highly.

Yogurt and Fruits

Yogurt is highly recommended for breakfast. It is absolutely forbidden to eat for dinner. You may have a breakfast of fruit and yogurt, but avoid taking hot drinks with them as they are antagonistic to each other. You may take your hot drink half an hour before breakfast. Avoid eating anything sour for breakfast, as sour disturbs pitta if eaten in the morning. Morning fruits should be bananas, papayas, or other sweet fruits, but not the fruits of citrus variety. Avoid readymade fruit yogurts; instead make your own fresh yogurt or buy just natural yogurt and add fresh fruits yourself. That way you can avoid consuming excessive quantities of sugar. Consuming too much yogurt may make you sleepy, and is not good for working efficiently.

Note: People with a weak digestive system should avoid yogurt. If you have aches and pains, avoid yogurt during that time period. Preferably, eat only freshly prepared yogurt. Yogurt that has turned sour should not be eaten.

Lunch or Dinner

When a meal is balanced with all the rasas, it is an Ayurvedic meal. If you eat the right amount of food, this meal will not make you feel drowsy at work after lunch. It is important to eat some grains with vegetables.

Simple Vegetarian Plate

Take 3 tablespoons green peas
1 medium-sized carrot
1 potato cut into small pieces
1 chopped onion
1 teaspoon finely chopped ginger
3 tablespoons finely chopped spinach
2 teaspoons of ghee or cooking oil

Add all the ingredients to a frying pan and cook for about 10 minutes while stirring. After two minutes add $\frac{1}{4}$ teaspoon spice mixture containing cumin, anise, fenugreek, and kalonji. Add salt to taste. Preferably, use a mixture of rock and sea salt. Serve either with cooked rice or one or two toasted slices of bread according to your need. Some cress salad or chicory to accompany this will make it a perfect meal. End the meal with something sweet, such as a light fruit, some cottage cheese, or any other dessert made of milk or cheese but not from grains.

COMBINING FOODS

I have provided a simplified list of foods earlier (Table 2, page 119), dividing them into three categories—cold, hot, and balanced. If you find that your favorite food is not balanced from the Ayurvedic point of view, but yet you want to eat it, as it gives you tremendous pleasure, you can create a balance by adding some simple spices. If, for example, you are eating foods from the "cold" list which I have specifically marked as "vata," cook it with plenty of ginger and some garlic. I highly recommend the use of ginger. The use of spices may be new to some of you. The specifications given below will provide you with guidelines. I also suggest that you prepare some spice mixtures that you can use regularly to make your food revitalizing. Instructions to cure diminished humors with specific nutrients are given in the last chapter of this book.

The following list of herbs and spices is essential for Ayurvedic cooking. They are easily available at Indian shops that cater to the needs of Indian immigrants abroad. These shops are easily found in big cities but even small towns are beginning to carry exotic herbs. Check your phone book for herb stores or Indian ethnic food. Some products are available at health food stores because so many people are eating a vegetarian diet.

Buying spices: Except for curcuma, which is difficult to grind, buy all other spices as such, and make powders yourself. Make sure that the spices are not too old as they lose their properties with time. In some supermarkets, the spices are very old because they do not sell quickly. Use a small stone or clay mortar or even a small coffee grinder for making powders for cooking or using spices as medicine. Once you have ground the spice, you can store the powder in tightly capped jars.

Ajwain: Ajwain seeds smell like thyme. Ajwain is available at Indian shops. If you do not happen to have it, you may replace it with thyme. However, thyme is milder.

Anise: Anise seeds, which look like cumin but are bigger in size and greener in color, are available almost everywhere. Fennel is a similar plant but it does not taste as nice in food as anise does because its seeds are harder.

Basil: Basil has become very popular in the West now, thus it does not need much explanation. The variety available abroad is milder than basil in India. I suggest that you keep always a green basil plant in your kitchen as it is used for both food and medicine. It is known to enhance the body's immunity. In case the green plant is not available throughout the year, you can use dried basil leaves, but be careful that they are not more than two months old.

Cardamom or Small Cardamom: This is well known as simply cardamom. I write it as "small cardamom" to distinguish it from another Ayurvedic plant product known as "big cardamom." Thus, the small cardamom is not different from what you simply know as cardamom. It is even available in supermarkets. Buy the greenish variety and not the white one.

Big Cardamom or Greater Cardamom: This is different from small cardamom in its looks as well as properties. Despite the similar name, you **cannot** replace them with each other as they are very different in their properties. The small cardamom brings the three humors into balance, whereas the big cardamom is pitta-promoting. Big cardamom is an excellent medicine for curing low blood pressure (see the last chapter of the book). People with hypertension should avoid it.

Big cardamom is about three times bigger in size than the small cardamom and is brown in color. It is available in Indian food shops.

Clove, Cinnamon, Pepper: I guess that these three do not need much explanation as they are used very commonly almost everywhere in the world. Cloves are the buds from a tree which are plucked at that particular state and dried. Cinnamon is a bark of a tree. Pepper is the fruit from a creeper. White pepper is made by taking out the husk of the ripened fruits of the black pepper. This way, it becomes less pungent.

Coriander: Coriander seeds are used as a spice and they are easily available everywhere. Coriander can be grown in pots; the leaves are used to flavor salads. Seed powder is used in cooking.

Cumin: Be careful when buying cumin as you should not confuse it with *carvy*, which has properties different from this cumin. It may be marked as white cumin (direct translation from Hindi) in some Indian food shops. For us, cumin is a spice, whereas *carvy* is used generally in medicines.

Curcuma: This is a root like ginger, but yellow in color. It is also known as turmeric. It is generally available in powdered form. Curcuma has a very strong yellow color, therefore be careful not to stain your clothes when you use it as either food or medicine. Curcuma should be put in hot oil or ghee before you add the rest of the food when you are cooking. Or, you can cook it in water for a long time, as when making soups, lentils, and so on. You cannot add it to the dish at the last minute because of its strong taste and flavor.

Dill: In the West, people know dill as an herb. The seeds are used in Ayurvedic cooking as well as in medicinal therapy. Dill is available at health food stores.

Fenugreek: Seeds are used as a spice. Fenugreek is available at health food stores. Its sprouts can be used as a salad or a vegetable. Its Indian name is *methi* or *methe,* and in Indian shops you can also buy its dried leaves.

Ginger: The use of fresh ginger is recommended in cooking, but in some recipes, one has to use dry ginger. It is suggested that you should keep both on hand.

Kalonji: These are black, tiny seeds of triangular form, rounded at the base. Erroneously, kalonji is sometimes called black cumin. In India, carvi or caraway, which is actually a variety of cumin, is called "black cumin." There are some people who confuse kalonji with onion seeds. Therefore, be careful when buying this spice. In Indian shops, the herb is marked kalonji even though it may be translated as "black cumin" in English.

Mustard: Mustard seeds are used in Ayurvedic food and in medicinal therapy. They can be obtained from Indian shops as well as from the health food stores. Tender fresh mustard leaves can be used as a vegetable.

SPICE MIXTURES

You may use your spices just as they are or as a combination of one or two, but it is also convenient to have some spice mixtures on hand. When you are a beginner with Ayurvedic cooking, these mixtures are more convenient and make things easy. Make small quantities of the various mixtures—a six month supply. As you know, ground spices lose their value more quickly than the seeds.

Spices should be well cleaned before they are put in bottles for use, or made into powders, as sometimes you'll find small stones or other dirt in them. Ajwain needs to be washed and dried. Put it in water, the stones or earth will settle down, whereas the ajwain seeds will float. Fish them out with a strainer and wash them a second time in a similar manner. Then put the ajwain on a linen or cotton napkin and spread it with your hands so that it can dry. Make sure that it is completely dry before you put it in a bottle.

The powders of the spices should not be made very fine, as they will lose their flavor quickly. They also taste better when they are kept a little granular, like sand. I will describe three mixtures, but you can make your own mixtures according to time and need.

Spice Mixture 1

Coriander, 1 ounce (25 gm)
Anise, 1 ounce (25 gm)
(or mix any equal quantity)

Clean the spices well. Grind them with your coffee grinder (or mortar and pestle), and put them in a bowl. Stir well so that they mix properly. Store the mixture in a clean, dry jar and mark it Spice Mixture 1. This mixture is "cold" in nature and will serve to balance all those foods which are "hot" in nature.

Spice Mixture 2

This is a rejuvenating mixture that you can use from time to time. Do not use it all the time as you will get tired of the same flavor; nevertheless, use it often!

Coriander, 2 ounces (50 gm)
Anise, 2 ounces (50 gm)
Cumin, 2 ounces (50 gm)
Ajwain, 2 ounces (50 gm)
Ginger, 2 ounces (50 gm)
Clove, 1 ounce (25 gm)
Cinnamon, 1 ounce (25 gm)
Pepper, 1 ounce (25 gm)
Nutmeg, 1 ounce (25 gm)
Fenugreek, 1 ounce (25 gm)
Big cardamom, 1 ounce (25 gm)
Small cardamom, 1 ounce (25 gm)
Nutmeg flowers, $\frac{1}{3}$ ounce (10 gm)

Clean all the ingredients; dry them by either putting them in the sun briefly or place them in a lightly heated oven for about half an hour. Grind them with the coffee grinder (or mortar and pestle) and put them in a big bowl so that you can mix them properly. Store the mixture in a clean, dry jar. Label it.

The dose per person in a meal is $\frac{1}{3}$ to $\frac{1}{2}$ teaspoon.

Spice Mixture 3

In this mixture the spices are not ground, but just mixed.

> Kalonji, 1 ounce, (25 gm)
> Cumin, 1 ounce, (25 gm)
> Fenugreek, 1 ounce, (25 gm)
> Coriander, 1 ounce, (25 gm)
> Anise, 1 ounce, (25 gm)
> Mustard seeds, 1 ounce, (25 gm)

After cleaning the spices well, put them in a big bottle so that it is only half filled. Shake the bottle until the spices are thoroughly mixed. Label your jar. This spice mixture is in balance and promotes strength. It has to be put in hot oil or ghee before you add the other ingredients to be cooked. If you are cooking in water, you can put them directly in the water.

Dose per person in a meal is ¼ teaspoon.

You may use other combinations of spices according to your discretion and need, but keep in mind their effect on you. Always consult the tables where I have classified them according to their "hot" and "cold" properties. Take into consideration all the ingredients you are using in a meal and their Ayurvedic nature.

I have given Spice Mixture 1 to be used with "hot" foods. For "cold" or vata-promoting foods, you should always think of using ajwain, garlic, and/or fenugreek. Spice Mixtures 2 and 3 will also help bring equilibrium.

GRAINS AND LENTILS

Here I specifically mention three kinds of beans that are especially important in Ayurvedic cooking. They are also a good source of protein for vegetarians.

Massor beans: These are available in Chinese and Egyptian food stores, as well as in some supermarkets. They are generally eaten without their skins and are pink in color. They are vata-promoting but pacify pitta. They are taken with ghee for pacifying pitta.

Mung beans: These beans can be cooked with or without their skin. Without skin, they cook quickly and are easier to digest. Both types are available in Indian or Chinese food shops or health food stores. They have a dark green skin and are yellow inside. Mung beans are known for balancing the three humors and therefore it is a good strength-promoting food when one is unwell or feels weak.

Urad beans: Urad beans look the same as mung beans, but the outer skin is black. They take a long time to cook. They are available only at the Indian food shops. Urad beans are well known aphrodisiacs (see the last chapter). Contrary to mung beans, these beans are strongly kapha- and pitta-promoting, and should be avoided when you are unwell, as they are heavy to digest.

6

PRAKRITI—THE BASIS OF
UNDERSTANDING AND HARMONY

IN CHAPTER 2, I talked about prakriti, or your fundamental nature. Your appearance and personality traits reveal your prakriti. You know that you should eat and live according to your prakriti, and the balance you try to maintain at the physical level through these multidimensional efforts helps keep your mental balance as well. I have described the fundamental role of prakriti at an individual level up to this point.

This aspect of Ayurvedic wisdom can also be used at a group level. We can create a productive and harmonious atmosphere at work by working with this energy. Personality clashes decelerate efficiency and create an unpleasant atmosphere. If you pay attention to the people you work with, if you try to understand them from their fundamental nature, you will be able to build a working group that is based upon understanding and sympathy for each other. You can also hire people according to their suitability and capability to work at a particular job. You can also match people up so that their character type works with the group. You can avoid a tremendous amount of clashes and irritations on the job, which means that you will end up liking your job and going to work. Let's see how this works in practice.

PRAKRITI AND BEHAVIOR

We sometimes hear older people commenting affectionately upon certain reactions and behavior of their middle-aged children by saying, "He is just the same as he was during his childhood." And couples often try to change each other for the "better," hoping the partner will change personality. Ultimately they give up their effort, saying, "I have given up, he or she will never change."

If you look around you, or observe yourself, you will realize that there are certain ways of acting and reacting that always stay with you. For example, you react in a particular way—whether it is the doorbell, telephone, or replying to a question. If you react quickly, you will do so all your life if you are a vata-dominant person. In normal conditions (non-pathological), the personality traits of vata-dominant people are a part of their being until their last days of life. Similarly, to have slow reaction times and responses, an inability to make decisions quickly, or postponing things to the next day, are traits of kapha-dominant people. You cannot expect these people to become like vata people, as their fundamental nature is part of their being. Those who are generally impatient by nature cannot delay their meals, and if they have to, they get angry and irritated—the pitta-type.

The above described traits are a part of the prakriti, or the fundamental nature, of an individual. The qualities for this way of behaving have been there since birth. As I explained in chapter 1, all living beings are a combination of body and soul. The soul is an energy without any substance; it is the cause of consciousness. The material body is made of five elements. As soon as the five elements come in combination with the soul, there is a living being, and there is a need for performing all the basic bodily functions. This task is done by the *doshas* or the three humors. In other words, the three humors are formed from the five elements, and that is why I think that the most appropriate translation of the *doshas* is the "three vital forces of the body" rather than the humors.

KARMA AND PRAKRITI

Let us look at some profound aspects of prakriti in order to understand what is predetermined and what we can do to change ourselves. According to Charaka, prakriti is determined by the constitution—the sperm, ovum, uterus, and the food and be-havior of the mother, time, and the *mahabhutas* (the five funda-mental elements).[1] These are the circumstances of one's birth. Who determines the circumstances of our birth? Prakriti, or even vikriti (as some people are born with an imbalance of the humors and are not healthy at the time of birth) comes from the previous karma of an individual, and from the previous karmic connections with other people which bring him or her into a particular birth situation. The sum total of all previous karma is called *samskara*, and it is due to your samskara that you behave in a particular manner or have specific interest from childhood. However, this does not mean that you are con-demned with a particular future. Your freedom lies in your sense of discretion with which you are able to continue your karma further. This means that you have the freedom to im-prove upon the results of the past deeds. The Ayurvedic term for the results of previous karma is *daiva*, and present karma is *purushakara* (see note 4 of chapter 1, page 7). For good health, harmony, and peace you need to find a balance between your daiva and purushakara.

Your daiva provides a certain terrain and it is with personal effort—or your present karma—that you build your present and future. The people you work with form a kind of karmic group, even though you each react differently on the job, and come from different families and social status. In big cities like Paris, London, Berlin, or New York, people who work togather come from different ethnic groups from all over the world. To bring Ayurveda to the workplace, you need to consider karma. If you understand your karma, you can bring peace and harmony to the group, and learn to work efficiently together. When you work well, you will stay healthy because you won't be irritated by your coworkers!

Let's see what measures you can take to promote this under-standing and harmony. When I talk of harmony, please under-stand that it is important to have harmony with the nature of your work, the place where you work, and the group of which you are a part.

---

[1]Charaka Samhita, Vimanasthanam, VIII, 95.

UNDERSTANDING YOURSELF

It would be nice if everyone in the work group made an effort to understand his or her constitutional type. That probably won't happen. But it is essential that you attain an awareness of your own habits and behavior in reference to your prakriti if you are going to take charge of your life. Only then can you realize the flexibility you have within a given framework. If you learn to know yourself in reference to your prakriti, and learn to observe your actions and reactions minutely, you will also be able to observe others in the same way. This process will help you see yourself without excessive involvement, for with the fundamental philosophy of prakriti, you begin to realize your limitations, and begin to comprehend that the time is not limited to one lifespan or to the short limits of your memory.

With this wisdom, you also learn to observe others within their limitations and with more compassion and sympathy. Despite the limitation of your fundamental nature, each of you, with your present karma, can keep your balance and can attain inner peace and harmony. Peace and harmony in a particular work atmosphere has to start with each of you individually. Then you can open up and deal with your relationships with the other people around you. Knowing where you fit in is one of the most important things you can bring to a job. You can really change your circumstances by taking the time to do this.

I am sure that you have figured out your fundamental nature or prakriti. In the present context, it is important to analyze your behavior and reactions so that you can make those changes for the better. Also keep in mind that prakriti changes into vikriti and during the vikriti (non-health) cycle your behavior may be different. You may be stuck in a vikriti mood for a long time, and in that case, it's important that you don't confuse your "normal" prakriti with vikriti.

Suppose your life gets very hectic, you have problems getting enough sleep, you keep yawning during the day, and you are making impulsive decisions. This is a state of vikriti. It is quite possible that you are a vata type and you have vata ailments because vata is diminished. There is also a possibility that your prakriti is not vata, but is due to an excessively vata life-style. In chapter 2 I said that you should recall your behavior and reactions during childhood to determine your prakriti. In any case, whether your prakriti is the domination of the same humor that is out of balance, or you have vikriti due to another humor, you should, first of all, bring yourself back to a state of health.

Let's imagine that you are a healthy person with vata prakriti. You are efficient and quick at work but when there are vata weather conditions, like strong winds, or you didn't get enough sleep, or you were at a party until late at night, or you ate the wrong food, your vata vitiates. In this state, you become confused and nervous, get impatient and easily irritated, and make impulsive decisions. This kind of energy doesn't support efficiency as far as your job is concerned. You have to learn to observe these factors and should take the necessary steps to stop yourself from doing this to your body. On this theme, I have said enough throughout this book. In addition, you should be conscious of the fact that when you are not working at your best you should avoid making important decisions. You should be able to analyze your faults and flaws and try to see them in perspective.

For example, as a writer, if I discover either through students, or on my own, that I have made a mistake or have written instructions in an unclear manner so my students could not understand what I was trying to teach, I examine the circumstances in which I wrote that particular copy so I can identify the factors that influenced my work that day. Was it an angry telephone call that I received while I was writing and which ultimately proved to be a hindrance in my communication? Was it vata vitiation, or the excessive Delhi heat? Why did not I keep my sattva state for doing my work? Analyzing the past will help us to correct ourselves, preventing similar mistakes in the future.

You all know that there are certain days when you feel that nothing goes as it should. You are not productive in terms of your work and you are also not in a particularly friendly mood. There are some situations when you understand that and say, "Well, because I was up late last night, or I did not digest my food properly, or I did not sleep very well due to some reason, and so on." There are other times, when you say, "I do not understand why I am like this today." Women may experience humoral changes during one menstrual cycle and because of that, their behavior may vary. There are also multidimensional factors, which may lead you from the state of health (prakriti) to non-health (vikriti). This affects your work as well as your interaction with others. When you know you are out of balance, you should try and use all the rational methods to come back to the state of health, and on this subject, there are instructions throughout this book.

The other way to deal with the situation is at the mental level. You should always try to do your best, even when you are out of balance: and this is possible through a sattvic mental state. When you do not feel in tune with your surroundings, and you have some subjective symptoms of not being well, directly or indirectly, you may bring negative energy into the workplace. You may also begin a chain of problems at work, and may not understand any direct cause for them. You all experience days when you end up saying, "Nothing works today!" At these times, it is the calmness and stillness of your mind which can help or hinder you from beginning a chain of negative reactions.

The moment you are aware that you are not in an optimum state, you can evoke your spiritual energy to help you in this difficult situation. Spiritual energy is a source of energy that lies dormant within. When you temporarily shut your senses to the outside world and stop this chain of thought, you evoke this dormant source of energy. In fact, the energy of the soul is not really "dormant," in the literal sense of the word. This energy is always radiating from the soul, but worldly activities—which are dominated by rajas and tamas—make a blanket of darkness around the spiritual energy and hinder its path. When you silence your mind using personal effort and various yoga practices, the blanket of darkness disappears and you will be guided by energy from the soul. With the help of this energy, the tamasic qualities (anger, irritation, jealousy, intolerance, etc.), disappear and you are able to express the qualities of compassion, love, tolerance, and so on.

With some easy to do exercises, you can make an effort to evoke your sattvic energy to hinder negative traits which may be due to a temporary state of vikriti. (See the breathing exercise on page 137). However, every effort should be made to attain a state of prakriti from vikriti. Following are some immediate measures that you may take if the various humors are out of balance. In case of vata vitiation, try to get immediate relief by drinking something hot, by massaging your ears, or by sending the prana to your head region. In the case of pitta vitiation, drink cold water or some other cooling drink, apply sandalwood paste to your forehead, and send prana energy to your solar plexus. In the case of kapha vitiation, try to do some vigorous movements or fast walking, and do the rapid breathing exercises (page 68) explained in the pranayama practices in chapter 4, page 66.

SATTVA FOR BALANCE AND HARMONY

Sattva not only helps you develop positive qualities during the state of vikriti, but also to bring balance and harmony in everyday life. The qualities of tolerance, love, and compassion help enhance mutual understanding and support in a group. These qualities are necessary for enhancing efficiency in a group on the one hand and in individual creativity on the other. The moment you are angry, irritated, or dissatisfied, you will make mistakes no matter what the nature of work is. One mistake leads to another and creates a vicious circle of irritation and anger.

What I mean to convey here is that you should develop the sattvic quality of your mind even when you are functioning in total balance. There are certain things in each of the seven types of prakritis that "we tend to do." That means that each prakriti has certain specific negative tendencies, such as anger, irritation, lethargy, intolerance, dissatisfaction, and so on. These traits may not come to the surface in normal circumstances, but in a given situation, they may be evoked in you. Even in specific and provoking circumstances, you should make an effort to keep your equilibrium by evoking sattva (fig. 35, page 138). I include some simple practices that might be helpful in this direction.

Breathing and Concentration Practices
to Achieve a Sattva State of Mind

1. Breathe deeply and send prana energy to your solar plexus. Let it stay there as long as you can while concentrating on the

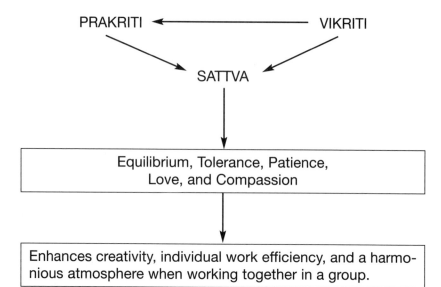

Figure 35. The state of vikriti can be changed to prakriti by using sattva-enhancing techniques.

plexus region, as this is the site of the soul. Exhale slowly and smoothly. When all the air is out, hold the lungs without air while continuing to concentrate on the solar region. Repeat this three times. At the end of each breathing exercise, pronounce the mantra "OM shanti" (universal peace, harmony, and stillness).

2. Do the same exercise again, but this time send the prana energy to the head region. Repeat the "OM shanti" mantra the same way. Do this three times.

3. During this last and third exercise, send the prana energy to every part of your body. The energy should flow in your head first, then in your arms up to your hands, to your thorax and abdominal region, and through the legs until it reaches your feet and toes. Hold your breath and exhale slowly and smoothly, visualizing the flow of energy all over in your body. Repeat this three times and remember to pronounce the "OM shanti" mantra each time.

These exercises involve breathing nine times. You may also take additional breaths in between. Including all, it should take you not more than seven minutes.

UNDERSTANDING OTHERS

After you have trained yourself to observe your actions and re-actions in the context of your fundamental nature or prakriti you will also begin to know vikriti behavior. It is natural to see other people in the same perspective at this point. It's a good idea to cooperate with the people you work with based on the context of their fundamental nature. For example, if you are a vata personality and you work with someone who is kapha, don't get irritated at the slow pace of this person. Learn to have patience, and think about the slow and steady progress this person can make while you forge ahead. There are other reasons why people don't work at your pace. Maybe your coworker has personal problems. Imagine one of your colleagues, someone who is dreamy and absent-minded, who seems unhappy, who is definitely inefficient at work. You are often irritated by this person. One day you learn from another employee that this person used to be very efficient at work and always had a happy disposition. Two years ago, she lost her 12-year-old child in an accident, and ever since this person is no more her usual self. After having learned this tragic story, your attitude toward your colleague changes and you become more understanding and sympathetic. In a similar manner, you can try to comprehend others who may have past life circumstances in their special context even if you do not know about it. In a working situation, if you all try to understand each other's reactions, a feeling of togetherness develops, and the group functions at a more personal level. This will inspire you to help each other, and to have compassion and love for each other.

My practical experience shows that the advantage of understanding others in the context of their prakriti is that people are not so self-involved, and are not embarrassed, touchy, or sensitive about accepting their so-called negative traits. The group learns to understand that specific personality traits are linked with physiological reactions and behavior patterns, and pointing these out is not passing judgment. Neither do people feel helpless, as they realize that there is a way to change themselves that requires a change in attitude or a change in nutrition.

To illustrate my statement, let me give you an example. Normally it is difficult to point out people's personality traits in a group seminar. However, when I teach the three humors and how they work at the level of body/mind, the students themselves begin to point out their characteristics and admit their specific traits. They do not try to justify themselves, or prove that their anger is caused by other people's behavior, etc. When I say that kapha people postpone their work until the next day, or that they are daydreamers or lethargic, people accept it easily if they happen to fall in this category. They feel very enthusiastic about the fact that they can do something to alter these characteristics by changing the food they eat and adding some specific yoga exercises to their daily routine, etc. They no longer have the impression that body/mind are two separate entities, or that they are responsible for their reactions when they really need dietary guidance. In a way, using the Ayurvedic wisdom of prakriti and the personality types, the fundamental feelings of guilt and self-blame are taken away. People get a new sense of freedom, and can begin to recognize their own characteristics and those of others.

Knowing each other's prakriti can help you deal with interaction with others on the job. Everything has a time and place. For example, you never ask questions of a pitta person or discuss other work problems just before lunch. These people cannot tolerate hunger and are easily angered immediately before meal time. Also watch your interaction with pitta people when they come inside after having been out in the hot sun. Vata people are easily exhausted in windy weather. Therefore, let them relax a little when they come to work when the wind is blowing. Rainy, cloudy, dark winter days tell upon kapha people, and if you want to have an important business meeting with them, invite them for a hot and spicy meal.

Some basic training in Ayurvedic wisdom can initiate a successful process of mutual understanding. People are usually intrigued with this way of thinking, for it is so different from the mechanistic way of looking at the universe, body, mind, personality, and behavior. Making a few simple adjustments can help create an atmosphere that is more human and loving, and which gives rise to more productivity and creativity in any business situation.

PRAKRITI AND TEAMWORK

People who are involved with management can pay attention to these Ayurvedic principles so that they place the right people in the right places for efficient management and productivity. In this direction, they should look at people's prakriti before hiring them for a particular job. For example, kapha people don't work well at night; pitta people will not do well on field jobs in hot countries; vata people do not work well outside in cold climates. Jobs where patience and tolerance are required will be more suitable for kapha types. Pitta people are not generally suited for such jobs. Vata people will do best where quick reactions are part of the job description.

When hiring groups, management should avoid putting too many people of the same type together. An all-vata group may create confusion; add some kaphas to bring balance. Too many pittas together, especially during the summer months, may end up generating anger. An exclusive group of kaphas may make for a lethargic atmosphere where nothing gets finished quickly. Thus, to avoid storm (vata), fire (pitta), and flood (kapha) situations at the work place, it is best to mix the different prakritis. On the other hand, when people work in pairs, do not combine vata and kapha, for vata and pitta will be much more creative.

SELECTING PERSONNEL

Observing the prakriti of new employees can be very beneficial. It can help you see, in addition to technical qualifications, whether or not the personality is suitable for the kind of job you are offering. For example, a job that involves a lot of travel will not be suitable for kapha types as these people are essentially home loving people. They may accept the job and assure you of their suitability, but there is a probability that they may develop a sense of frustration that will eventually affect job performance. Pitta people may not be suitable for retail sales management because of their impatience. Sales may be more suitable for kapha people for they have more patience and tolerance. These two qualities, patience and tolerance, are extremely important when dealing with the general public.

There are many things that we bring to a job interview when we are looking to hire a new person. The people hiring should know the nature of the job, the details of the job description, and the rest of the staff the person they are hiring will be working with. It is also important to know how to judge the candidates by external appearance and outward behavior. Complexion, eyes, nails, and hair will show many characteristics for classification. Additional information comes from the way people talk and react in conversation. Kapha people may be slow to react, but they generally will not misunderstand your statement, which vata types might tend to do. Fine-featured pitta types may show impatience—through facial expression—by the time you reach the end of a long sentence, or if you talk about some aspect of the job too long.

SELECTING PROFESSION
ACCORDING TO SAMSKARA AND PRAKRITI

It would be helpful if parents observed their children carefully and paid attention to the interests that "come from within them," so they could help the children select their profession accordingly. We all have different *samskara* and thus different prakriti. Parents and children or siblings may not have the same professional interests. It is not uncommon to see that two siblings have quite opposite interests and choose professions in entirely different fields.

Parents should not impose their own ideas on the choice of a profession for their children. Values like "family honor or prestige," or simply the "convenience factor" about an already set up profession compels many parents to impose a profession on their children. Due to this, not only do these individuals suffer all their lives from being in the wrong profession, but the damage is paid in much larger sums than that. It affects our whole society as people in the wrong profession will perpetuate their frustration on the job. Their basic dissatisfaction will also influence their relationship with the people with whom they interact. In fact, this is a very crucial subject. As an employer, you want to hire people who will be happy and productive.

7

SATTVA—
A KEY TO EXPAND TIME

THE DIFFERENCE BETWEEN the holistic and the mechanistic approach to work is that in the former, everything is interdependent and interrelated. That makes the holistic system sound complicated, but the approach is very logical. If we compare the human body to a machine, its systems seem very simple as long as we forget about consciousness. For human beings, machines are simple because people have made the machines themselves and can understand them. However, human beings are far more complicated than any machine. Machines work on command and do not have consciousness. Human beings have a sense of discretion or intellect (buddhi) and due to that they have the faculty to decide things for themselves. That makes the interaction between human beings very complicated as compared to a computer network.

It is not possible to use holistic medicine without living a holistic way of life, and it is not possible to lead a holistic life only in private, as it touches all aspects of your existence. You cannot ignore your work situation, personal relationships, social behavior, or sexuality, and if there is an imbalance in one of these, it slowly affects the other aspects also, and a chain of negative events begins. The holistic system opposes chance theory and emphasizes that nothing happens without reason.

According to the mechanistic approach to life, chance plays a great role in cosmic events and human life. Influenced by this view, many people live very fragmented lives. They are supposed to do their work in a way that is organized more or less like a machine, and, after all, there is this general belief that there is only a material reality. Thus the existence of soul as the cause of consciousness is not recognized. The concept of the dormant spiritual energy that lies within all of us, that is evoked through *sattva* (see also the preceding chapter), and that can be used for a beneficial purpose, is not accepted by this mechanistic view of life. Actually, the absence of this inner stillness and peace and other related sattvic qualities is the cause of many evils and ailments.

Due to the imposition of the mechanistic view, our lives are extremely imbalanced and are dominated by rajas and tamas and there is hardly any sattva. In chapter 1, we discussed the six-dimensional equilibrium human beings should try to maintain. All six dimensions are interconnected and an imbalance in one of the six gradually causes an imbalance in the whole life.

People are always "in a hurry." Time is very well planned— sometimes a year, two years, or even several years in advance. Once, when I was on holiday on the island of Bali, I met a woman from Switzerland. She commented that, "People in Bali think that we Europeans are very happy and fortunate as we are rich. They do not know that we work like crazy and we can never lead the relaxed lives they do on this island." Indeed, this is very true! I feel the same when I go to our Himalayan center from Delhi. People living in the interior of the Himalayan mountains have simple but tranquil lives. Each time, when I return to Delhi, in contrast, I see the predominant madness due to awfully "busy" and stressful lives of people around me.

In the rajas-dominated lives, there is also a substantial amount of tamas. Modern life is full of competition. And people are not honest when they work. This takes a toll on each of us. A salesperson, for example, has to give false arguments to convince people to buy the product being sold. The big business houses tell many lies to sell their anti-health, anti-environment products. A farmer spoils the earth with pesticides and industrial chemicals affect our water. Life is full of rajas and tamas. There is a lack of sattva. There is no stillness and peace in the real sense. People are too busy, even during their holidays, which are again rajas-dominated. Daily leisure time is mostly rajas. Watching television is generally rajas and tamas and disturbs vata and kapha if too much time is spent looking at the screen.

People go on with a daily routine predominant in rajas and tamas, with equally rajas-dominating leisure time. The daytime is rajas and the night is tamas. During the night, they go into a tamas state of mind as sleep is tamas. However, due to the hectic activity of the day, their sleep is also intermingled with rajas. Then the next day begins and they again live in a state of rajas mixed with tamas. Life goes on like this until there comes a day when some of them cannot take it anymore. After a long hyper-rajas period, some fall into a predominating tamas state. That means that they end up depressed, or become prey to another serious ailment. It is absolutely essential that we organize our lives better and intermix our activities during the day and sleep during the night with sattva to create a balance. If we are able to bring a balance with sattva in the rajas and tamas aspects of our lives, we will be able to work with a calm mind, we will feel rested, and will be able to withstand pressure at work. If we are able to draw energy from the immense source (the soul) with sattvic methods, stress or tension generated at work will not affect our health. Similarly, with our efforts, if we are able to get sleep that is also sattvic, we will be rejuvenated, waking refreshed from a great night's sleep. The 16-minute program (page 76) is meant to bring sattva in your work and sleep time.

For longevity, health, and better productivity, sattva is an asset. If you train the mind to obtain inner stillness, you are able to accomplish more in less time. In addition, sattva is essential to keep balance in the three activities of the mind, for without it we gradually create a humor imbalance as well. Let us see how it happens.

Excessive rajas gradually leads to vata imbalance. It also leads to sleep disturbances, which is an activity of vata. At the mental level, excessive rajas or too much activity during the day should be balanced with calmness and peace; and if this is not done, restlessness is transferred to sleep time. This means that the disturbances, tension and confusion of the day need to be brought to a stop with conscious effort. Otherwise, you go to sleep because you are physically tired, but your mind is not at rest. Or, if the nature of your work is such that it does not physically tire you, you may not be able to sleep.

If you are a vata-dominant person, not sleeping well may cause constipation the next day. The constipation will further diminish vata and you may feel tired and stiff upon getting up in the morning a day later. You may also feel restless during the night and have a dry throat. Thus, a series of events are initiated with an imbalance in one of the six major factors responsible for the body/mind activities and for the qualities of the mind. In fact, due to the predominance of rajas in our modern way of living, vata is the most easily diminished humor of our times. I often say that we live in a vata civilization. By bringing sattva into our daily lives, we can also prevent this humor from vitiation and can avoid health problems. Let us see how we can integrate the sattvic way of being.

SATTVIC PRINCIPLES IN DAILY LIFE

In order to strengthen the sattva quality of the mind, you have to get rid of fear, grief, greed, and confusion. Fear and greed lead to other negative qualities, such as jealousy, excessive attachment, possessiveness, and dissatisfaction. All these qualities hinder the way you do your job as well as making you unhappy in other areas of your life.

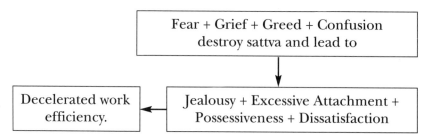

You have to make a conscious effort to get rid of these negative traits. You should try to think about the impermanence of your existence. You should enjoy every minute of your life as much as you can. Even if you are unhappy for one reason or another, some beautiful things in this fascinating world should cheer you up. A singing bird, a tree in bloom, the setting sun, the stars, or the moon should fill you with joy. Moments gone never come back, it is up to you how you spend them. If you lament over what you don't have or what you could not get, you destroy a substantial part of your life. Live in the present moment and do that particular thing you are supposed to do in that given moment—whether it is your work, or driving your car, or eating your food, or taking a bath, or anything. Whatever you are doing, do it with perfection, give it your best, not only with your mind but also with your heart.

To the rationalists, the Cartesians, and all those believing in the mechanistic view of life, this statement may sound ridiculous. But when a meal is cooked with love and affection, it tastes better—delicious as compared to when it is mechanically done. That is why so many adults all over the world never forget "what their mothers used to make for them." In Ayurveda, there are specifications for making medications. It is advised that you make medications in a peaceful mental state while chanting mantras and stirring the herbs in a specific manner. All this increases the healing qualities of the medicine. Thus, in this specific example, you see that when you are totally involved with the act you are doing, you not only perform the act better but also enhance the basic value of the product in terms of benefits.

Let's look at how you can learn to be completely involved in what you are doing in a given moment of time. In Ayurveda, there are a number of rituals and ceremonies that can be used to develop awareness of the body, cosmic changes, major life events, your work, the economy, traveling, and so on. I have tried to simplify some of them so that you can adapt them to your modern life-style.

Before I proceed further, I would like to add that sattva is not exclusively in Ayurveda or in the Indian tradition. In former times, religion handled this role. In almost all religions, there are prayers before meals, before bedtime and before traveling. There are churches near seaports and railway stations. Somehow, when they built airports, they did not build places of worship, but prayer rooms are now being made available to travelers.

I have already talked about sattvic activities in this book. For example, the 16-minute yoga program is geared toward that, and some words before beginning your meal have the same purpose. In Ayurveda, it is said that each time you leave the house, you should touch either a godhead or a deity or a precious stone. I suggest that, whatever the object you choose to use, concentrate on that. Pray that you will return home safely. It only takes a minute and it sets the mood for the day. So, before you begin your journey to work, pray that you are safe on the road, in your car, or whatever the case may be.

I suggest that each time you put the key in your car, you make the similar wish for safety. Place an OM or a picture of a saint or spiritual leader in your car to seek the blessings each time you begin a journey. However, if you do not want to do that, at least make a wish for health and safety when you drive. You may also breathe deeply and make a *kavacha* around you as I explained in the chapter on yoga (see pages 68, #5 and 99).

When you begin your work day, pray for a good, productive, and peaceful day for yourself. Do not begin your work abruptly or in a huff. Similarly, when you end your work day, do not rush, give some thought to how your day was and whether you are happy with what you've done and give a moment to the atmosphere at work. If you didn't have a good day, then wish for a better next day and make an effort for that. This concept applies to anything you do. You can do the same when you cook, or when you undertake any new project or program.

I am not suggesting that you lose time in all these "thoughts," or that you should work slowly. Actually, you don't need any extra time to begin or end your work days peacefully as I have suggested. It is just the matter of training your mental state.

Being totally involved in what you are doing helps bring consciousness to your state of being. That means you don't work like a robot any more for you are conscious and aware of what you are doing. This is helpful in developing your mental faculty, for when you work in a mechanical way, you end up behaving like a machine. Secondly, when you work with self-awareness, your productivity goes up as your intuitive faculty becomes more active. You become more creative and work at a more profound energy level—which is sattvic. The sattvic state of mind is closer to the soul. It is through sattva or the stillness of mind that a yoga adept reaches the pure state of consciousness and becomes one with the cosmic energy.[1]

---

[1]Refer to my book *Yogasutras of Patanjali: A Scientific Exposition* (New Delhi: Clarion Books, 1996). See Part I, Sutras 3 and 4.

In former times, religious or folk festivals were used to celebrate the change of season. These festivals were often associated with the harvest. In addition, there were many elaborate ceremonies to mark the major events in life—weddings, pregnancy, childbirth, a new house, and so on. People still celebrate some of these events even now, but generally they have a party. The customs and rituals which had a profound symbolic significance and that prepared people psychologically for these major changes, and helped them to concentrate their mental power for these events, have been lost with modernization. We need to bring back some of these festivals that highlight principal events in a more spiritual way for the rituals provide us with mental strength. We can use some significant mantras, or we can concentrate on the mountains, rivers, stones, sun, moon, or other sources of energy to highlight any new beginning. We need benediction, for it evokes spiritual energy. We can seek these blessings from holy persons or from natural cosmic energies.

In other words, we must learn to develop a relationship with time. In the Indian tradition, time has tremendous significance in all respects; time is considered "holy." It is venerated in the form of goddess Kali. *Kala* is time and *Kali* is the goddess of time. We Hindus specifically pray to Ma Kali when we need time to finish a specific project so that we get enough physical and mental power to finish in the time allotted. There are many direct and indirect ways of evoking spiritual energy. We can use certain breathing techniques to make a protective armor around us. We can concentrate on the solar plexus before beginning a new project. All these help bring us above the material level that generally revolves around material existence.

CONTROLLING
EXCESSIVE USE OF THE SENSES

I have already explained that the sattva state is achieved by stilling the mind. By bringing the continuous chain of thoughts in your mind to a standstill you are able to evoke the immense source of spiritual energy within you. If you are excessively indulgent in the activities of the world, the inward path to this energy becomes difficult to find. If you are immersed in the activities of the five senses, and even when you sit to do breathing exercises or concentration practices, it becomes hard to concentrate. To enhance the quality of life, for longevity, for increasing productivity at work, and for developing creativity, it is essential to refrain from excessive use of your senses.

You need to use all your senses constantly; the only time the senses temporarily cease activity is when you sleep. This temporary cessation is actually only partial, because loud noises, too much light, or very strong smells, will wake you up. Sleep provides tremendous rest after a day's activity and rejuvenates you for the next day.

When you do exercises to attain mental concentration (popularly known as meditation), you consciously withdraw your senses and try to concentrate your mind on a single object—like a mantra, or a part of your body, or anything else—you are able to refresh yourself mentally and physically in a very short time. It takes less time to rejuvenate via meditation than it takes to do the same thing from sleeping. Why? Because you withdraw from rajas and tamas and go into a state of sattva temporarily. That means that you enter the state of pure consciousness where "I" as a person no longer identifies with the senses, but with "my" soul, which is the cause of consciousness. If you concentrate briefly on your inner being, it saves you from fatigue, it enhances your work efficiency and leads toward sattva. I will explain this statement with various examples.

Some people talk all the time at work. This sense is associated with the sense of hearing. You can exercise restraint in the use of these two senses by gradually training yourself to speak only as much as you need to. Learn to be precise and avoid senseless conversation. If your job involves a lot of speaking, you need to create a balance with some quiet time in the evening when you don't have to talk or listen. If possible, find some quiet moments during the day in order to create an equilibrium. Take a deep breath and send the prana energy to your mouth, tongue, throat, and ears. Even it it's only two or three breaths a few times a day, this practice will help keep inner peace, and will make you aware of your talking activity.

I have noticed that people who talk a lot also watch a lot of television in the evening. This leads to an excessive use of the sense of hearing. The mind also gets hyperactive. While they are young they can handle the pressure, but after age 45, the over-stimulation begins to tell upon them. Thus, for stable health, long life, and good working capacity, it is better to create an equilibrium than to use the senses excessively.

In some work situations, like with computers, photography, working with microscopes and so on, you use your eyes all the time. You should also try to do the breathing exercises mentioned above. This time send prana energy to the eyes and the region around the eyes. Make sure that, from time to time when you do not require your sense of sight, you give your eyes a rest by shutting them. Find some time in the evening to lie down quietly and shut your eyes. It will be helpful if you can put a cold wet compress on your eyes from time to time.

It is not possible to go into details of all the specific senses that people might be using in excess during their work day. My basic message is that we should pay special attention to our bodies and notice what we stress, and in addition to the many rational methods of healing discussed in the chapter on yoga, we should energize the overstressed parts of our bodies with prana energy. Excessive use of the senses or other particular organs of the body can make us restless and becomes a hindrance in the path of sattva. If you intersperse work time with an effort to get sattvic energy to create balance, you are able to work better. In a way, this small investment of a few minutes—in terms of the breathing exercises—brings heavy returns in the form of working time saved by enhancing your efficiency.

DEVELOPING STILLNESS OF MIND

The earlier discussion about controlling the excessive use of your senses is, in a way, preparatory to this next step, where you learn to develop stillness of mind. I have noticed that the Western style of teaching meditation, doesn't work because it is not taught with the proper techniques. This means that people study it and then don't use this asset. You need to learn appropriate techniques. With regular practice, you will develop enough self-control so that you are able to spontaneously achieve the state of mental stillness. But if people are not taught that the first step is to learn to restrain their senses, meditation becomes simply sitting quietly in a group. It does not help in any way for anything.

There are a number of very specific and simple techniques that will gradually lead you to experience your inner wealth. These techniques are based upon the authentic source of yoga, *The Yoga Sutras of Patanjali,* mentioned earlier. However, these techniques should be followed after an appropriate preparation with yoga postures, breathing exercises, and self-restraint over your senses. You should also keep in mind that if you want to achieve success, you need to do the concentration exercises regularly. If you make very little progress—like about 0.25 on the scale of 10—and discontinue the practice in between, it is quite possible that you might have to begin from zero again!

These techniques will help you develop spiritual energy, thus enhancing your intuitive capability. This latter is beneficial for developing mental faculties, creativity, and talent. The capability to evoke dormant spiritual energy and to be able to live on a more profound plane of consciousness is an asset in every walk of life.

I have described four different techniques for achieving the stillness of mind popularly known as "meditation." It is suggested that you begin with the first technique and then move on to the others. You may finally keep up with either the third or fourth technique. Those of you who already have some experience may begin directly with the third or the fourth technique.

Continue doing the concentration practices described here, even if you only have a few minutes to spare during the day. Your spiritual energy is also like the other forms of energy—you have to get it constantly in order to have its benefits.

The First Technique—Japa

This technique is called *japa,* or the repetition of a mantra or a word. It is especially beneficial if you have difficulty in silencing your mind after the day's hectic activity. OM is the smallest mantra, and symbolizes the Universal Soul or the cosmic energy (fig. 36). You may choose some other rhythmic lines or words, or

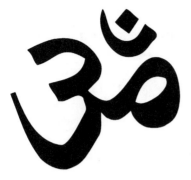

Figure 36. The figurative form of the mantra OM, symbolizing the Universal Soul.

some other mantra, or another word. You may have heard group singing, where the group repeats the same mantra or a line of poetry. This is called *keertan*. Singing keertans is a very helpful practice to silence the mind. I always do this practice in my seminars and it is very successful. My students do not understand the meaning of the Sanskrit words I give them, but the rhythm becomes very important and helps to bring the mind to stillness. Unfortunately, the theoretical explanation of japa is not enough in this case and perhaps in future, I will try to make an audio cassette for those who cannot be in the seminars. I suggest that you join a group to do this kind of singing, for it opens a path to sattva for all of you. (There are keertan tapes available from some specialist groups; check your metaphysical bookstore or any of the ashrams in your area.)

The Second Technique

This practice of silencing the mind involves exciting one of your senses to the utmost, for then you reach a state of stillness automatically. We do this practice in our Himalayan center by taking a bath in very cold Ganges water and then using the spiritual energy for healing. But the sense of touch is not exclusive for doing this practice. There are ways to evoke other senses for this purpose. A very strong taste can excite your sense of taste and serves the same purpose. I am sure that all of you have had this experience at one time or another in your life. When you eat an extremely spicy meal, for a few moments, the spices can make you forget everything. In the present context, the idea is to prolong this thought-free state of mind. You may do this with your sense of smell, by smelling something intense and pleasant-smelling. Have you found yourself getting lost while inhaling a sweet-smelling flower, or while looking at a beautiful sunset, or while listening to some exquisite piece of music? It is the similar idea that is the basis of this concentration practice. It is done with the aim of prolonging that moment when you are with nothing else in your mind but this one specific sensation.

The Third Technique

This technique involves learning to concentrate on a single external object. That means it is external to your body. Let's use a tree as an example. Sit down in a relaxed posture, close your eyes, and visualize internally the image of a tree, preferably a tree you actually know well and see often. If you wish, and if it is possible, you can actually look at this tree before visualizing it with closed eyes. Once you have the image of the tree in front of you, think about why it is called a tree. You will realize that the name as it sounds has hardly any significance, as a tree is called different names in different languages, but a tree is a tree because of its specific characteristics. A tree is called a tree because of the testimony given to this particular name with those particular characteristics. Thus, you begin to concentrate merely on the form of the tree. That means that you get rid of its name, the logic behind its being a tree, and you stay only with the form of the tree as you perceive it. Try to concentrate just on the form of the tree.

After a few days of regular practice, you may feel that you are completely able to concentrate on the form of the tree without the other thoughts entering into your mind. At this stage, try to forget even the form of the tree, just realize only the essence of it. Concentrate for several days until you experience a oneness with the essence of the tree.

The Fourth Technique

In this technique, concentration is focused on one of the internal parts of the body. It may be on the tip of your nose, the place between your eyebrows, the lower part of your throat, your solar plexus, and so on. These places are the sites of the energy chakras.

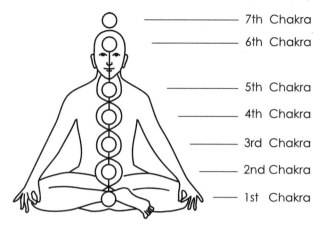

7th Chakra

6th Chakra

5th Chakra

4th Chakra

3rd Chakra

2nd Chakra

1st Chakra

Figure 37. Circles of concentric energy or chakras in the body.

The chakras are the sites of concentric energy where the three major energy channels of the body cross each other (figure 37). In the present context, I suggest that you concentrate on the solar plexus or on your forehead between the eyebrows (the third eye). Choose your place of concentration and do not change it again and again. To visualize the image of OM (see fig. 36, page 155) at the place of concentration will be helpful to achieve success. You may also visualize the sun. But the image of the sun or OM is to be in that limited place where you are concentrating. The image provides support for the initial stages of concentration. However, later on if you are successful, the image disappears automatically and you remain in contact with only this limited space of your body. This state may be short-lived, but with repeated practice, you will be successful in prolonging it.

THE SATTVIC WAY OF DEALING WITH OTHERS

When you begin the concentration practices, you will automatically adopt other sattvic ways that provide you with extra energy and the ability to sense events and other things before they happen. In other words, your "inner voice" will develop and will show you the way to make the right decisions at the right time. A sattvic way of life also helps you overcome tamasic qualities, such as fear, greed, jealousy, and so on. You will develop kindness and compassion, which will enhance your cooperation and understanding of others. Of course all these are not achieved in a day, and these qualities grow as a result of the constant effort you put into this development. Therefore, when you have begun the concentration practice, also develop the other allied qualities—self-restraint and being kind and understanding to others. Try to have patience and tolerance for others.

However, this does not mean you should not be assertive wherever necessary, or that you should be over-indulgent with others at your place of work. In fact, many people misunderstand the real sense of compassion. It neither means pity nor does it mean to take over other people's pain; it is to understand their problems well and help them find a way for themselves. If this quality is cultivated at your workplace, your strength and compassion will enhance cooperation and the spirit of teamwork.

What I wish to convey in this section is that each of you should try to be understanding and patient with the other people you work with—to be as accommodating as you can. Sattvic goodness is not for ego satisfaction; it is without selfish motive, and it is also without a mercenary attitude. You are not being good for the sake of others, but for yourself. You are finding your own way, which pierces the cover of darkness from your soul and shows you the spiritual light.

In a diplomat's house in Delhi, I read a placard saying, "Diplomacy is when you can say to someone, 'Go to hell,' in such a way that the person actually looks forward to the trip." Sattvic dealings are not much different from this. But here, the power of convincing should come from your own spiritual strength. It requires a tremendous amount of humility and patience. But if you follow the sattvic practices described above, these qualities become a part of your spontaneous behavior.

In the previous chapter, I explained how you should try to understand other people according to their prakriti. Here I emphasize that you should also engage in sattvic behavior with others. Try to forget and forgive, and always look forward to a better relationship in future. This will help you get over trivial differences and create harmony in a pleasant work environment.

RELAXING TENSE WORK ENVIRONMENTS

Despite all your efforts, it is quite possible that differences may arise and an atmosphere of tension take over the workplace. There are times when rational talking does not help ease the group tension, and the more you discuss the situation, the more complicated it becomes. Sattvic singing (keertans) or silence is very helpful to release tension in such situations. You can decide mutually to forget the differences and make an effort to get on with life. Sattva teaches you to get rid of your ego and recognize your real self, the cause of consciousness. Thus, in such a situation, a short session of singing "OM shanti," or some other mantra, or simply doing the silent concentration exercise for five minutes may help you. Depending upon the situation, you may also want to try the laughing exercise (page 96) to bring the group to a happy mood. Or try the lion's cry (page 97) to throw away the aggression if any is left in members of the group. You may want to read chapter 4 on yoga again.

LEARNING TO WORK WITHOUT STRESS

Some years ago, a few young Germans (about 20 years old) visited me here in Delhi. Each time I asked them how their day was or how their visit to the museum was and so on, they always replied, "Good but stressful." Observing them, it seemed that life itself was a stress for these young people. Even after a trip to the Himalayan mountains, they replied the same way. It seemed that these young people had made "stress" their perpetual mental state; they were incapable of completely relaxing and letting themselves loose, or else they use the word "stress" to highlight the importance of their activities.

Stress is actually a mental state that does not bring anything positive. It is a kind of pressure we exert on our minds which is rooted in fear and insecurity. These two tamasic qualities eat up our energy and take away our time. Instead of enjoying life (as in the above example) or working, our energy is used up with stress.

If we are short of time and there is plenty of work, we need to concentrate with all our might to finish that work and not to waste any energy in stress. Stress hinders our capabilities and thus our output diminishes. Stress is something we should always save ourselves from as it is tamasic and destructive.

Sometimes you need to finish a certain piece of work to make a deadline. That is where you need sattvic energy. You should do some concentration exercises before beginning the job and seek the blessings of the sun or the moon to give you the ability to finish the project in the given time. Breathe deeply, and send prana energy to the solar plexus in order to inspire yourself. This inspirational energy is within you. You must be able to distinguish a stressed mental state from the state of mind that is totally engrossed and devoted to doing a particular job.

In a seminar on work efficiency, an executive of a multinational company told me that in one of the seminars given by an American teacher, he learned that a certain amount of stress is necessary for working efficiency. I don't agree with this view at all. As I said earlier, stress stems from fear and insecurity. Perhaps fear makes you work faster. It could also be that the fear of losing your job, or the fear of not earning enough to meet expenses, or the fear of displeasing your boss, might be the basis for your stress. But sooner or later, stress will tell upon your health. On some people, its effects are seen fairly quickly, but there are others who tend to accumulate stress. This latter situation is worse because it gives rise to mental or physical ailments that erupt like a volcano when the stress level becomes too high.

With sattvic methods, you learn a dimension of time that is different from the time told by the clock. When you work with spiritual energy, you are able to expand time as you get more energy and creative power by evoking the dormant spiritual energy within you. To develop enough so you can take advantage of this inner "abundance energy," you have to invest devotion and determination.

8

PROMOTING STRENGTH
AND PREVENTING ILLNESS

THERE IS A state of body and mind that falls between health and sickness. I discussed this theme in chapter 2 and called it a state of "non-health," known as vikriti. The state of non-health is due to an imbalance of the three vital forces of the body, or it could be due to low vitality and immunity. Our efficiency at work is diminished more due to this state of non-health than due to serious ailments. People are physically present on the job, and function just enough to be there, but they are not strong and healthy enough to do a great job. In fact, this prolonged state of non-health gives rise to more minor ailments which result in more loss of productivity and more absence. Keeping all this in mind, I will deal with three principal themes in this last chapter. First, the diagnosis and cure of humoral imbalance; second, enhancing immunity and vitality; and third, some suggestions for warding off ailments.

THE DIAGNOSIS AND CURE
OF HUMORAL IMBALANCES

Despite all the care and attention you give to keeping your balance nutritionally, as well as living with natural rhythms to maintain the balance between the three humors, and the three qualities of mind, from time to time, you are still going to be subjected to an imbalance because of circumstances. For example, if you have to travel for a long time, or you stay up too late at night, or eat a meal that is not exactly suitable for your constitution, an imbalance may occur. You should be able to detect the effect of this imbalance, diagnose it, and cure it immediately. It is easy to cure minor health problems at the initial stages. Later, when a humor has been vitiated for a long time, the negative effects seem perpetual and chronic troubles set in. Keeping this in mind, I provide cures using simple home remedies and allied precautions.

For a Vata Imbalance

Here are some examples of vata vitiation so you can use this wisdom spontaneously. Let's say you had to stay up very late at night for some reason. This disturbs vata. To save yourself from this imbalance, eat warm and fatty foods that are balanced from the Ayurvedic point of view. Don't forget to drink hot water when you get up the next morning, so that you don't get constipated, for this usually happens after a sleepless night. Use ajwain, ginger, fenugreek, and cumin in your meals, or simply drink a tea made from ajwain, thyme, ginger and basil. (See recipe on page 164.)

It is also quite possible that a situation might occur when there is more than one factor that disturbs the function of a humor. For example, you have to travel for many hours on a business trip and finish working on a project that keeps you so busy you don't even get time to have warm meals. In addition, the weather is very windy and your hotel is on a noisy boulevard in a big city. Here, you get a package containing everything you need to throw your vata out of gear. Obviously, the effect is much greater if you are a vata-dominant person. The intensity of the humor imbalance will depend upon your vitality (*ojas*). The time it takes to cure the problem will depend upon the measures you adopt. In any case, in this example, when you are facing multiple factors that contribute to vitiate the humor, you need more intense treatment than in the first example.

Dill seeds and garlic are two more substances that cure both vitiated vata and kapha. Promote their use in your food, or take them as medicine, but do not exceed the prescribed dose.

$\frac{1}{2}$ teaspoon dill per day

2–3 cloves garlic (medium-size) daily

Dill oil may also be used; its dose is 1 to 3 drops per day.

½ teaspoon cress seeds or ½ teaspoon fenugreek per day are the two other remedies to cure vitiated vata and/or kapha.

Remember that to cure vitiated vata, foods with sweet, sour, and saline rasas should be used. Pungent, bitter, and astringent nutrients should be avoided.

In all the herbal remedies described above, the substances involved are "hot" in their Ayurvedic nature. Thus, you can have side-effects in terms of pitta imbalance, especially if your prakriti is pitta. Generally these side-effects are observed in terms of an excess of heat in the body. Hands, feet, or the head may become excessively hot and you may experience excessive sweating. Some people get pimples in some part of the body, or you may get a blister in your mouth. To save yourself from these side-effects of the treatment, take 1 teaspoon anise per day. Either chew it or make a cold decoction from it (see recipe on page 164). Or else, you can choose to eat those fruits and vegetables which are "cold" in nature so that a balance is created.

Coming back to the example when you risk vata vitiation with multiple factors, you must also learn other methods to bring back your balance. In case of a high degree of vitiation, drinking the above-mentioned teas may not be enough. First of all, it may take time to restore your balance. After a few hectic vata days described in the above example, you must compensate with some rest and peace. If you continue to go out every day after you worked very hard, and then to also have a week-end full of activities, the vitiated humor either vitiates more or continues to remain imbalanced. In the beginning, symptoms like a stiff body, some aches here and there, a dry throat, etc., may be tolerable, but gradually, when they become a regular feature, you begin to feel fatigued and exhausted. You need to have an oil massage, and should take both types of enemas described earlier. Along with this treatment, you'll need the above-mentioned teas, as well as hot meals with ginger, garlic, and spices. A hot bath, appropriate rest and a peaceful atmosphere will help restore the vitiated humor. You will find that, with these treatments, your body will get rid of the negative symptoms you were experiencing due to vata vitiation and you will feel energetic and rejuvenated. You may not notice this so much when you are very young, but when you are over 40, you should really allow yourself some time to rest and relax.

Ajwain, Thyme, Ginger, and Basil Teas

All these teas are of a "hot" Ayurvedic nature, and are helpful to bring vata and kapha equilibrium in the body.

Ajwain tea:	Boil 1–$\frac{1}{4}$ cup (250 ml) water Add 1 teaspoon ajwain Let water boil covered on a low fire for about 10 minutes.
Thyme tea:	Boil 1–$\frac{1}{4}$ cup (250 ml) water Add 1 teaspoon thyme Let water boil covered on a low fire for about 10 minutes.
Ginger and Basil tea:	Boil 1–$\frac{1}{4}$ cup (250 ml) water Add 1 inch (2–3 centimeters) cube of ginger in crushed form Add 5 fresh basil leaves (or $\frac{1}{2}$ teaspoon dried leaves) Let water boil covered on a low fire for about 10 minutes.

Filter this tea with a tea strainer and drink it hot.

You can use crystal sugar to sweeten the tea, but remember not to use any honey as it is antagonistic to heat. It is never to be heated above 95° (35° C) which means that you shouldn't use honey in hot drinks or in baked foods.

A minor imbalance of vata will be cured by taking this tea once or twice daily for two to three days.

Ajwain or thyme tea is excellent to get rid of hangovers. It is suggested that people who drink alcohol use this regularly.

Cold Decoction from Anise

In Ayurveda, it is said that some substances are sensitive to heat and lose their medicinal properties if heated. They should be taken in powdered form or soaked in water at room temperature for several hours. Anise is one of these substances.

To make a cold decoction of anise, soak 1 teaspoon anise in a ¾ cup (150 ml) glass of water and stir well with a spoon. Cover and let it steep for at least 4 hours or overnight. In case you need the decoction quickly, make it with powdered anise and stir it vigorously in water. Then let it steep for at least 15 minutes so the powder settles down. In both cases, you can filter it before drinking. If you don't filter it, and if you chew the seeds or eat the powder, this is also all right and even more effective.

This decoction is also used to cure diarrhea. Take the same dose three times a day.

For a Pitta Imbalance

Some of the minor but nagging ailments caused by a pitta imbalance are blisters in the mouth or on the tongue, heat in specific parts of the body, reoccurring digestive problems, rashes, acne, burning sensations in certain parts of the body, tearing and thickening of the skin, excessive perspiration, unpleasant body odor. One or more of these problems can be easily cured by bringing this humor in balance. Let's see how we can cure these ailments and appease the excessive fire in the body.

The excessive physical fire is brought under control with sweet, bitter, and astringent rasas. If your prakriti is pitta, remember that you must always include these rasas in your food and lessen the use of sour foods. Eating sour foods during pitta vitiation is like adding fuel to the fire. Hot food with chilies and an excess of salt have a similar effect. You cannot always live the way you are supposed to, and driven by circumstances and desire, you may get sidetracked from your path. First of all, you should take care that this diversion should not be excessive, and you should not stray from the path too often. Second, when you do not live according to your prakriti, you should learn to take quick action to fix the problem. When you have eaten an excessively sour, rather salty and pungent (with chilies or other spices with a similar effect) meal, you should compensate with a big fruit salad (exclude sour fruits), or a glass of cold milk, or drink an anise decoction. Drink plenty of cold water, and take a cold shower or bath if the weather permits. See page 166 for some other simple measures to regain pitta equilibrium.

If there are several factors at once which vitiate your pitta strongly, you would need to take several steps to bring this vital force back to its normal function. For example, if you happen to be in the hot sun on the same day, and you also eat salty, sour, and hot food with chilies, drink some alcoholic beverages, and happen to have a situation that makes you angry, the accumulated effect of all these may be strong, and the above-described mild measures may not be enough. Then you need to take purgation therapy, a cold bath, and massage (anointing) with pitta-decreasing substances. This latter is particularly beneficial if pitta is diminished in specific parts of the body. See page 167 for external applications of pitta-reducing substances.

Substances to Balance Pitta

Wormwood: This plant is well known in the West. Its leaves and flowers should be used. You can make a decoction by putting 1 teaspoon in 1 cup (200 ml) boiling water. Let it steep for about 10 minutes. Filter it and drink it. Since this tea is very bitter, you may find it unpleasant to drink. Alternatively, you may make a powder of the leaves and flowers and gulp it down with a glass of water. Take $\frac{1}{4}$ teaspoon of the powder. The precise daily dose is 1–3 gm per day.

Endive: Powdered seeds or root should be taken. The dose is $\frac{1}{2}$ teaspoon daily. Gulp down the powder with some water.

Coriander: The dose of powdered coriander is $\frac{1}{2}$ teaspoon daily. The decoction may be made by boiling the powder in 1 cup (200 ml) of water for 15 minutes, covered, on a low fire. The powder can also be consumed straight with water.

Neem: This is a very effective medicine to cure pitta and kapha vitiation. Take either 5–10 drops of the oil daily by putting it in some water (about $\frac{1}{2}$ cup or 100 ml) or make a decoction of leaves and bark. You may take the powdered leaves and bark as such. The daily dose should not exceed more than $\frac{1}{2}$ teaspoon. The decoction should be made as it is described for coriander.

Massor beans: Cook the beans ($\frac{1}{2}$ cup or 100 ml) in 2-$\frac{1}{2}$ cup ($\frac{1}{2}$ liter) of water for about half an hour. Add more water if needed so that it looks like a soup. While it is cooking, add $\frac{1}{4}$ teaspoon anise seeds, salt to taste, and $\frac{1}{4}$ teaspoon curcuma. When the soup is ready, take it with 2 to 4 teaspoons ghee. The quantity of ghee depends upon your digestive capacity. Take this preparation as a soup.

Massage to Pacify Pitta

If you have a burning sensation in some part of the body, or a feeling of excess heat, or too much perspiration, you can use one of the following measures:

1. Coconut oil or ghee are two cooling oils which can be used to massage the whole body. The head may also be massaged with these oils.

2. Sandalwood paste is very effective in curing external pitta vitiation and it also removes bad odors from the body.

There are two ways to prepare sandalwood paste. You may buy powdered sandalwood and make a paste with water. It is better to extract the liquid through a muslin cloth so that you do not get wood fibers on your skin. A better way to make the paste is by taking a piece of sandalwood and rubbing it on a rough stone (fig. 38, page 168). Add a few drops of water and rub the wood on the stone. Using your finger, wipe off the paste that you make and collect it in a little bowl.

Smear the paste on the required places with your fingers (fig. 38). You may smear your whole body with this. It is good to leave the paste on your body for several hours if you can. In fact, your body heat will dry it up and it will fall off. You may need to repeat the treatment for several days depending upon the gravity of your vitiation. This treatment improves your complexion and gives a radiant look.

3. Mud Bath: Generally yellow, fine earth is used for this purpose. Make a thin paste in water and smear it on your body. After the mud dries completely on your body, wait for at least 15 minutes before you wash it off. Besides bringing the pitta into balance, this treatment makes your complexion smooth and shiny.

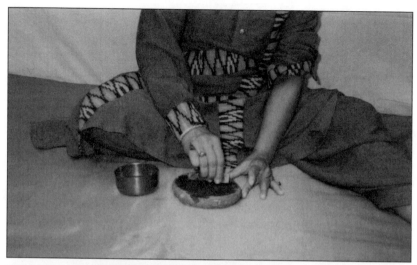

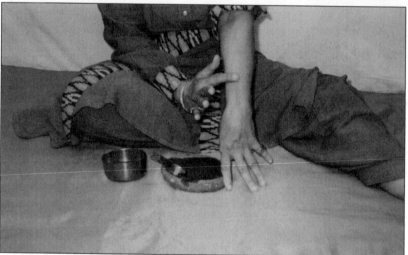

Figures 38. Top: to make paste of the sandalwood, rub it on a rough stone surface with water; Bottom: smear this paste on your body with your fingers.

For a Kapha Imbalance

If you are feeling lethargic and tired when you get up in the morning; if you feel like sleeping at work despite the fact that you had a good night's rest; if you feel heaviness in your body; if you realize that you have become slower in your actions; if you often get a sweet taste in your mouth; if you salivate excessively; if your body is retaining water; your kapha is vitiated. Depending upon the intensity of the problem, you may have one or more of these symptoms. Kapha, like the other vitiations, is your work enemy. In fact it is a stronger work enemy than the other two humoral vitiations.

With symptoms like these, don't think that you can cure yourself with rest. The more you sleep, the more you will be tired. On the contrary, make an effort to swing into action. You should never sleep more than eight hours. Do some physical exercise, go for a brisk walk in the mornings and evenings, and eat hot and spicy meals. Use plenty of ginger in your cooking, and also use the spices for vata wherever I mention that they are used for both vata and kapha imbalances. Be careful to use very little oil and reduce the sweet stuff. Avoid desserts made from flour or other grains, and avoid chocolate. Pungent, bitter, and astringent foods are used for kapha vitiation. Avoid sour, saline, and sweet. Pay attention particularly at dinner time. Do not eat late dinners, and avoid salt, especially at night. Try to go for a walk before going to bed. Remember that kapha vitiation enhances during the night when you are at rest and sleeping. It is contrary to vata which enhances with work and activity. To cure vata, a peaceful atmosphere and rest is necessary, whereas to cure a kapha vitiation, you need to enhance physical movement.

Hot baths and wet fomentations are of tremendous help to cure the vitiation of this humor. I have described fomentation, or the sweating treatment, in chapter 3. Here I will describe specific treatments using medications (see page 170).

It is quite possible that you may have kapha imbalance in a specific part of the body, such as water retention. In this case, a wet compress, pressure massage, and exercise of that specific part should be done. You will realize that the problems of kapha vitiation increase when you get up in the morning and during the day, they subside.

When kapha vitiation is too much and you are unable to cure yourself with these basic measures, you need to do emetic therapy. Take all the precautions and follow all the instructions given in chapter 3 when you do emesis.

It is quite possible that you can vitiate more than one humor. In the case of vata-pitta vitiation, you might get confused with the "hot" and "cold" substances to be taken. The substances that cure vitiated vata-pitta are anise and licorice. The dose and mode of consumption for anise is described above, and for licorice it is ½ teaspoon per day. Take the powder as such or boil in water for 10 minutes on a low fire and drink as tea. In vata-pitta vitiation, you need enemas as well as purgation and then begin with anise and licorice tea. Take one tea in the morning and one in the evening. Be sure to eat a balanced diet. Eat carrots, mung beans, mixed vegetables, and some rice. Also get enough rest and give yourself a coconut oil or ghee massage from time to time.

I have already mentioned many substances that cure vata-kapha vitiation. They both need warm therapeutic measures. You should take enemas as well as emetic therapy by following the instructions described in chapter 3.

For curing pitta-kapha vitiation, neem is excellent (for dosage and mode of intake, see the recipe on page 166).

If all three humors are vitiated, you need to do saptakarma, eat a balanced Ayurvedic diet, and use the medicines that create humor equilibrium. Turmeric, small cardamom, and coriander are medicines that establish equilibrium. Trifala, a mixture of three Himalayan fruits (amala, harad, baheda) is rejuvenating as well as establishing this humoral equilibrium. When all the three humors are vitiated for a long time, it is advisable to get help from an Ayurvedic physician or let yourself be treated properly with panchakarma or saptakarma therapy.

Wet Fomentations with Essential Oils or Specific Herbs

All substances that are "hot" in nature will be helpful to balance kapha. But you have to take care that these substances are also pleasant to the skin and do not produce an allergic reaction or cause irritations. A decoction of ajwain, thyme, or dill (4 ounces or 100 gm), or cinnamon (2 ounces or 50 gm), or big cardamom (2 ounces or 50 gm), or caster leaves (4 ounces or 100 gm) may be used for this purpose. Cook the chosen substance in 3 liters of water for about 20 minutes with the lid on. Cinnamon and big cardamom should be powdered before cooking. Remove the shell and powder only the seeds when you use big cardamom.

Once the decoction is ready, filter it and put small towels in it. Let them stay there for about a minute and then squeeze them with the help of a pair of big tongs (fig. 39). Make sure that the towel is not too hot for the skin when you spread it on your body (fig. 39). You can place a compress on your hands, feet, or other specific parts of the body, but for whole body fomentation, you will need the help of another person who will keep changing the towels and replacing them with new hot towels for you. You will need to heat the decoction once or twice during the process.

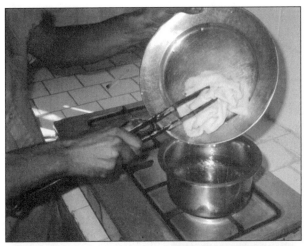

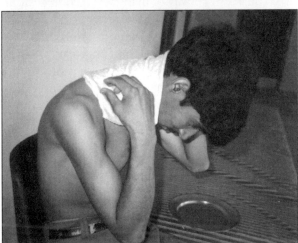

Figure 39. Top: wet compress to relieve pain. Squeeze the hot medicated water from the towel with tongs; Bottom: spread the compress over the affected part.

The use of essential oils in water is easier than preparing a decoction. Such oils are usually available in health food stores. You can also make your own combinations. A recipe for one such mixture is described in chapter 3 for doing head cleaning. You may use 1 teaspoon of this oil in 2 quarts of water.

Do not overdo fomentation as it causes weakness. Once you begin to sweat, stop it, cover yourself well and rest for at least 15 minutes. Make sure that there are no drafts where you do fomentation or rest afterward.

HUMOR IMBALANCE AND ITS CURE

Many people are now familiar with Ayurveda, and humor therapy is becoming very popular. However, there are times when the concept is not understood properly, and because of this lack of understanding, people misuse it. Rather than improving their health, they end up doing harm to themselves. This is due to the fact that Ayurvedic wisdom is taught by people who do not understand the fundamental basis and theory behind the physical and cosmic balances. Ayurveda is a health care system that combines medical, philosophical, historical, and traditional knowledge. To apply its principles to the Western way of living, we also need to understand Western life-style, nutritional habits, and cultural background. In order to impart the practical wisdom of Ayurveda in the West, the people who teach it must adapt the system to where it is being used. For example, an Ayurvedic teacher coming from South India, which is a hot country, may lay emphasis on coconut oil massage, which is not such a great idea for an American winter. Even in Northwest India we avoid using coconut oil in winter, and we use sesame oil instead. Ayurvedic prescriptions move with nature and differ considerably from the Himalayas to Sri Lanka.

According to these Ayurvedic principles, natural substances are neither good nor bad, and there are many external factors that have to be considered when thinking about appropriate nutrition and medication. By applying the wrong things at the wrong places and at the wrong time, we misuse these natural substances. This error is made because we try to use a reductionist approach to medicine, and we try to categorize life in a mathematical way. We think it is easier to label things as being good or bad. I have heard about many misinterpretations and misuses of Ayurvedic wisdom from my students in Europe. Therefore, I feel I must add some extra notes of caution from time to time.

The humors are not "three buckets of water" that should be equally full or equally empty to maintain good health. The humors are the vital forces of the body that perform all the physical and mental functions. If you have vitiation of a humor, you cannot simply stop eating the foods responsible for the condition to bring back vital force to the body. For example, if your kapha is vitiated, and you stop eating sweet, oily, and fatty foods, you will end up also vitiating your vata. You will become nervous and may have problems sleeping, you may be constipated, and you may experience other negative effects of vata vitiation. You may take this course of action because many Ayurvedic textbooks many teach that this is how you fix the kapha problem.

You must keep in mind that the humor vitiation is not necessarily an excess of a humor. It could also be its lack, or a humor is not in its place, or it is accumulated in one place, and so on. Thus, to cure vitiation, you need to work on a multidimensional level. Thus, it is quite a complex wisdom that should be understood and then followed properly in practice. This is the reason why, in this chapter, I am avoiding dealing with the theoretical details and giving you some very practical tips. Once you have practical experience, it is easy to understand the profound theory behind it. When European students come to our centers here in India, they actually "live" and experience Ayurveda. Most of them have read my books and have already attended seminars in Europe. They often comment that it is by experiencing through their own bodies that they actually understood the concepts intellectually learned earlier.

A NOTE OF CAUTION FOR USING NATURAL MEDICINES

Some people think that medications from plants are harmless, and they can take as much of it as they like. However, I have seen some people who took herbal medications in excessive quantities and created a humoral imbalance. Remember that everything you consume has rasas, and their basic elements will have some effect on your equilibrium. Many Ayurvedic home remedies are made from herbs and plants used in the kitchen, and higher doses are used as medication (see Curcuma Cure on page 104). If you take an excess of something that is "hot" in nature during the summer, it can cause too much heat in the body. You may experience pitta vitiation in one form or the other. When you eat too much of a food dominant in one particular rasa, and you eat it often, you may experience a side-effect in the form of humor vitiation. For example, if you eat a lot of sour food and you eat this kind of food frequently, you will get pitta vitiation. You may have any of the symptoms of pitta vitiation—indigestion, acidity, etc. Therefore, while curing yourself with natural medicines, respect the prescribed dose, the mode of consumption, specific combinations, quantity, and dietary instructions.

REJUVENATING THE BODY

It is important to eat foods that strengthen your immune system. These are called rasayanas (see chapter 5 for detailed descriptions of the rasayanas). Among the most familiar individual substances are basil and garlic. One makes a good rasayana when combined with several other foods. Here I am only working with home remedies; for other recipes, you may consult one of my other books, *Ayurveda for Life*. In the original Ayurvedic texts, there are many complicated rasayana recipes, as one of the eight parts of Ayurveda is about rejuvenation and longevity.

Rejuvenating Mixture
_____

    Anise, 2 ounces (50 gm)
    Licorice, 2 ounces (50 gm)
    Small cardamom, 1 ounce (25 gm)
    Big cardamom, 1 ounce (25 gm)
    Pepper, 1 ounce (25 gm)
    Ginger, 2 ounces (50 gm)
    Basil, 1 ounce (25 gm)
    Clove, 1 ounce (25 gm)
    Cinnamon, 1 ounce (25 gm)

Use dry spices. Clean them well; take the cardamom seeds out from their pods. Put all the spices together in a plate. Dry them briefly in the sun or in a warm oven to get rid of any humidity before you grind them in a coffee grinder. Do not grind them too fine; just keep them granular. Put the mixture in a bowl and mix thoroughly. Store the mixture in a clean dry glass jar with a cover.

Take $\frac{1}{4}$ to $\frac{1}{2}$ teaspoon of the mixture daily. Boil the powder in the amount of water you want to drink. Use a steel or glass pot; let the mixture boil (covered) for about 3 minutes and let it rest another 3–5 minutes. There is no need to sweeten it, as the anise and licorice make it sweet. You may take this tea either in the morning to get energy for the day's work, or in the evening to get over the fatigue of the day. You may also take this twice a day if you wish.

You may also make another recipe by adding black tea to the rejuvenating mixture. This makes an excellent, healthy tea for breakfast, which makes you active for the day's activities. Boil $\frac{1}{2}$ teaspoon of the rejuvenating mixture in 1 cup (200 ml) water for about 3 minutes and add 1 teaspoon granular black tea. Also add 1 teaspoon sugar (or according to taste). Let it boil for about a minute and add about $\frac{1}{2}$ cup (100 ml) milk and boil the mixture for half a minute. Strain and drink as a breakfast tea.

We don't recommend that you use this preparation with black tea after 5 or 6 o'clock in the evening as it (the black tea) can cause sleep disturbances even several hours after its intake. However, tea made from the rejuvenation mixture can be taken anytime.

This mixture is especially good to alleviate fatigue. It enhances ojas and protects you from minor infections. It increases energy and vigor and its regular use is recommended.

Preservation of Garlic in Honey

I have already talked about garlic being a rasayana in chapter 5 and have described how people should use it according to their prakriti. You can also preserve garlic in honey. According to Ayurvedic wisdom, the properties of many substances are enhanced when they are preserved in honey. Garlic is very heavy to digest and this preparation makes it easy to digest for people of all prakritis.

Take 4 ounces (100 gm) of garlic and peel the cloves. Spread them on a flat surface and let them dry for a few hours. Take a 16 ounce (500 ml) glass jar (with a cover) which is half-filled with honey. Add the garlic cloves to this jar and stir with a spoon so that all of the cloves are covered. Garlic floats in honey, so you have to push it down. Add to this mixture $\frac{1}{2}$ ounce (10 gm) cloves (clove spice, not cloves of garlic) and mix everything well. Close the jar and leave it in a dark cupboard. Open it every day and stir the contents, or shake the bottle to mix the contents well. It "matures" in about ten days and can be eaten.

You may eat 1 to 3 cloves a day, along with a spice clove. Begin with one garlic clove and increase the dose to three while making sure that you are digesting it okay. Normally, garlic in this form is easy to digest, but some people with low fire (poor digestive power) may have problems.

Take this rasayana in the evening so the smell is not offensive for others while you are at work. To get rid of the garlic smell, chew small cardamoms. In any case, chewing 3–4 cardamoms a day is a good habit to cultivate, as it balances the humors, perfumes the mouth, strengthens the heart, and makes the voice melodious.

Rejuvenating the Physical Fire

For good health and longevity, it is very important that we also rejuvenate the body's fire. The thoracic region of the body houses the lungs, heart, and liver. These three are the most vital organs in the body. The liver and other digestive glands also need rejuvenation from time to time, as their malfunction affects the whole thoracic region and ultimately the whole body. This is more important today than it was a hundred years ago because we are now subjected to various poisons in the form of fertilizers, pesticides, preservatives, and all kinds of chemical sprays in our food. These poisons gradually affect the liver and its allied functions.

I suggest that you take a liver rejuvenation cure at least once a year. The home remedy for liver rejuvenation may be taken for ten days after every six months. Those of you who drink alcoholic beverages often and in generous quantity should do this cure more frequently. Take wormwood, endive, or neem (described earlier in this chapter) regularly for ten days. During this cure, also drink ajwain and ginger tea once a day. Drink these two teas at different times, allowing several hours to elapse before taking the other tea. Follow the dose described for both ajwain and ginger. This treatment may cause mild diarrhea, which is a process of cleansing.

REJUVENATING BRAIN AND NERVES

Noise pollution and our hectic pace is very tiring to the nervous system, and it is important to revitalize the brain and nerves from time to time. After a lot of concentrated work, the head region may accumulate fatigue. Symptoms of this kind of fatigue are shown in the form of forgetfulness or "heaviness" in the head. I use a simple recipe to promote memory and strengthen the nerves. In Ayurveda, there are wonderful treatments and everything used in this recipe is easily available. It is recommended to take this tonic for thirty days. You may take this preparation more often, or even for fifteen days every month if you wish, for this tonic is also good for eyesight and promotes general strength in the body. If you want to be efficient at work, you must have a good memory, and therefore this rejuvenating tonic is important in the present context.

Brain and Nerve Rejuvenating Product

Cashew nuts, 2 ounces (50 gm)
Pumpkin seeds, 2 ounces (50 gm)
Anise, 2 ounces (50 gm)
Licorice, 2 ounces (50 gm)
Black pepper, 1 ounce (25 gm)
Small cardamom, 1 ounce (25 gm)
Honey

Take the cardamom out of their pods and weigh the seeds for the recipe. Grind the spices. Mix the powder well in a bowl and gradually add honey into it. Keep stirring so that it mixes well. Add just enough honey to make the mixture into a thick paste. Put it in a clean and dry jar (with a cover) and store in the refrigerator.

Take 2 teaspoons daily, as is, or preferably with warm milk for about a month. If you find that this tonic makes you put on weight, reduce the quantity to half or reduce your intake of other foods you are eating.

PREVENTING AILMENTS

In Ayurvedic tradition, there are three kinds of ailments. One category is innate; they arise from imbalances in different aspects of our life-style. We have discussed this theme at length and the main emphasis has been on creating a six-dimensional equilibrium so we can keep our mental and physical environment clean and healthy. When we do this, we will be happy, and happy people work efficiently for the well-being of our society.

The second type of ailment is caused by external infections attacking the body—such as bacteria, viruses, or even poisons and accidents. If we keep our humors in balance and take rasayanas so that our ojas are high, we will be strong enough to ward off or heal these external attacks. A mental state dominated by sattva also helps develop an intuitive capacity that enables us to avoid all kinds of accidents.

The third type of ailment is a psychic ailment that arises due to unfulfilled desires or having to face the undesired. Ayurveda advises that we develop sattvic values and follow a path of self-restraint, compassion, and tolerance. These values help us avoid this kind of ailment as we learn to control desires and understand the temporary nature of existence on this planet.

We prevent and create ailments through our karma, or our actions. For example, if we are careless and do not bother to maintain equilibrium in our way of living, we become prey to many disorders. If we still do not learn from this, the disorders slowly give rise to a serious disease. Life-long vata imbalance, which is symptomatically cured by taking chemical drugs for many years, may finally give rise to arthritis. Headaches or migraines are generally not cured with the remedies of modern medicine and are suppressed by strong chemical drugs. In fact, headaches and migraines are not even really ailments, but are a warning of a fatigued physical state and a blockage of the energy channels. Continuous use of chemical drugs to suppress these symptoms may give rise to stomach or kidney problems, or other side-effects. Then we take yet more drugs to cure these new disorders and get into the vicious cycle of disease and drugs.

There are some diseases that may be the result of past karma, and it is important to know how to handle them with our present karma in order to suffer the minimum. We cannot ignore our interactions with other human beings, for life involves a process of give and take. For example, when somebody close to us has a serious illness, we also suffer with this person. How we respond now builds present and future karma. We cannot change the karma we made in the past.

To adopt an Ayurvedic way of life requires time and attention, but it seems to be the only solution for preventing serious illness. Using the example of migraines once again, many people suffer from them and take strong drugs to avoid the suffering so that they are able to go to work. If they are taught Ayurvedic and yogic techniques so they can remove the root cause of this problem, they not only cure themselves without spending a lot of money, but they also avoid any related diseases that may occur later in the eyes, ears, nose, or the whole head region that would be caused as a result of suffering the migraine pain for many years.

Diseases like hypertension, diabetes, backaches, other aches and pains, cardiac ailments, sleep disorders, hemorrhoids, colitis, and so forth are virtually self-created because we don't know how to take care of our bodies. It is important for all of us that we pay attention to ourselves and spend some time on ourselves. We do devote time to ourselves, but it is mostly for decorating our external self with nice clothes and material possessions, or entertaining ourselves at a very superficial level. The fundamental wisdom of Ayurveda is very basic and deals with the simple facts of life. It teaches us to keep our body and mind in tune with the rest of the cosmos. If we follow this tradition, we will be able to live happier lives; we can be more productive at work, and we can give and share as members of a creative society.

Once in Varanasi (Benaras), I asked a vaidya (Ayurvedic physician) to check my pulse and diagnose my state of health. He replied laughingly, "I need not do so, as I am sure you have perfect health. It is because you are a prasanchitta person (a person with a happy and satisfied disposition)." Traditional Ayurvedic wisdom lays great emphasis on using a happy state of mind to prevent ailments, as well as for healing. Always make an effort to be happy. People are unhappy because they worry too much. They are afraid and insecure about the future. Fear is an enemy of health, while a contented mental state is health-promoting. We are worried and afraid because we believe in the permanence of life. We feel excessively involved in worldly things because we forget that we are here only temporarily. Things will work here even in "my" absence when "my" physical destructible being perishes—that being with which I identify myself. If we learn to enjoy and appreciate the small things of life, we can attain a happy disposition. The tremendous beauty of the cosmos can have a rejuvenating effect.

In the Bhagavad Gita, there is one chapter on karmayoga. The essence of it is that we should go on doing our duty (at work, in the family, and socially) with the best of our ability, with devotion, and without desiring results from it. With this devotion toward duty, we reach the status of a yogi. We should also recognize our duty toward body and mind mentioned in all yoga texts, because the path to salvation is through the body. The path to material fulfillment and worldly pleasure is also through the body, and therefore whatever our direction and aim, the body is the medium. Its care and protection should have the utmost priority.

Because so many people are interested in some form of spiritual growth, and because so many businesses are multinational— meaning that they embrace employees from many cultures and spiritual paths; and because so much money is wasted on health care that could be used elsewhere to solve world problems (of famine, for instance), it seems that using the Ayurvedic system in the workplace will go a long way to promote both prosperity and health on our planet.

OM SHANTI

GLOSSARY

anointing: It is called *lepa* in Ayurveda. Smearing the body with the pastes of different products (sandalwood, mud, oil, seeds or herbs) for creating equilibrium of humors and/or beautifying it.

asanas: Yoga postures.

basa: Foods that are either cooked well in advance, or preserved to enhance shelf life.

blood purification: Detoxification of the body by the intake of products or other methods.

dharana: Attention.

dhyana: Single-pointedness of the mind popularly termed meditation. In the technical sense, it is only a step to meditation.

emesis: Voluntary vomiting after the intake of fluids.

enemas: Cleaning the intestines with oily or non-oily liquids. Emesis and enemas are two of the seven purification practices.

five elements: Ether, air, fire, water, earth.

fomentation: These are sweat treatments done to remove toxins from the body. You can do dry fomentation, or wet fomentation. The wet fomentation is similar to a "Turkish bath."

fumigation: Another form of head purification by inhaling the smoke of burning herbs and performing breathing exercises.

hridya: Solar plexus where the soul resides.

jaladhauti: A yogic practice of cleaning the stomach by drinking salted water and vomiting it voluntarily.

japa: The repetition of a mantra or a word to attain a thought-free mind.

kapha: One of the three energies or humors responsible for the physical and mental functions of the body, the other two being vata and pitta. Driven by water and earth, kapha is responsible for the solid structure of the body.

kapha vitiation: Common cold, headaches, vision problems, loss of the sense of smell, taste, sinusitis.

kavacha: Spiritual armor.

keertan: Devotional chorus or group singing repetitive poetry or mantras with the idea of freeing the mind from worldly activities.

mahabhutas: Five fundamental elements: ether, air, fire, water, and earth.

nasya: Nasal passage.

nasyakarma: Purification of the head region by inserting medications through the nasal passage to revitalize the four senses and the nervous system.

ojas: Immunity and vitality.

panchakarma: The five purification practices; two kinds of enemas, emesis (voluntary vomiting), purgation (inducing diarrhea), nasya (cleaning the sinuses). Panchakarma preparation practices are called purvakarma.

pitta: One of the three energies or humors responsible for the physical and mental functions of the body, along with vata and kapha. Pitta is from the fire element and is responsible for digestion and body heat.

prakriti: Prakriti denotes the basic nature of the body which is to stay healthy. It is also the human fundamental constitution at the time of birth. It is determined by the quality of sperm, ovum, condition of the uterus, food, behavior of the mother, and other prevailing circumstances during pregnancy. The karma of the individual is another deciding factor regarding an individual's prakriti.

prana: Vital air.

pranayama: Breathing exercises.

preparation for saptakarma: Includes two kinds of unction (one body massage and ingesting oil to clean digestive tract), and fomentation (dry or wet sweat baths).

purgation: Creating diarrhea in order to revitalize the liver function.

purvakarma: Preparatory practices before doing panchakarma or saptakarma; includes massage, unction, and fomentation.

rajas: One of the three qualities of the mind which denotes activity, thinking, planning, making decisions, etc. The other two qualities are sattva and tamas.

rasa: Taste—sweet, sour, saline, pungent, bitter, astringent. There are six rasas.

rasayana: A substance, or combination of substances that invigorate the body and increase ojas (immunity and vitality).

samadhi: The third and last state of meditation, the first two being dhyana (concentration), and dharana (contemplation).

samskara: Sum total of all previous karma.

santosha: Contentment.

saptakarma: The seven actions or purifications, including two kinds of enemas, emesis, purgation, head cleaning, blood purification techniques and cleansing the urinary tract.

sattva: One of the three qualities of the mind which denotes peace, stillness, goodness, compassion, virtue, etc. The other qualities are rajas and tamas.

16-minutes-a-day: The first 3 minutes for morning breathing exercises; then 10 minutes for yoga exercises; the last 3 minutes for evening breathing exercises; done morning and evening for a total of 16 minutes.

sweat treatments: *See fomentation.*

tamas: One of the three qualities of the mind which denotes passiveness, inactivity, all that is counter movement and against development of the mind. Thus, qualities like greed, jealousy, pain, killing, etc. are also tamas qualities. The other two qualities of the mind are sattva and rajas.

unction: Body massage using olive oils and other oils, such as sesame or coconut oil or ghee. You can also use specially formulated oils (see recipes). *Also note:* Inner unction is done by consuming fat so that your body can attach toxins and wastes to the fat and eliminate them.

urinary tract purification: One of the saptakara purification practices which is done by taking strong diuretics once every six months to flush out all deposits and dirt from the urinary system.

vata: One of the three energies (humors) responsible for all the physical and mental functions of the body, the other two being pitta and kapha. Vata is from the elements ether and air and is responsible for all the functions of the body that are related to movements, such as, thinking, speaking, excretion, blood circulation, etc.

vikriti: State of non-health, impairment.

vitiation (of vata, pitta, kapha): Vitiation means a malfunction or disorder in the functions. One or more humors may vitiate in the body. Vitiation of a humor means one or more of the following: excess, lack, displacement, lack of coordination with time and space and the quality of that particular energy or humor.

DR. VERMA'S CENTERS IN INDIA

This book on Ayurveda is meant to be a very simple guide so that you can use Ayurvedic practices in your daily life. I encourage you to change your life by taking small steps—exercise you can do at home, remedies you can make at home, the 16-minute program, and so on. The herbs and spices introduced here are easily available. They belong to traditional Indian and Pakistani cuisine. I have tried to provide the Hindi names along with the English and Latin names for herbs and spices so you can locate them in Indian food stores.

Ayurveda is a complete holistic system of living and deals with all aspects of life. I am well aware that it is not easy to switch from a fragmented approach to a holistic one—either philosophically or in the various practical aspects of life. Therefore, I travel in Europe to give lectures, seminars and weekend workshops on "Ayurveda a Way of Life" and other subjects, such as holistic sexuality, Ayurvedic nutrition, stress management with yoga and Ayurveda, and so on. These can be organized by invitation and I am always in Europe between August and November of every year. I am happy to travel to the United States to lecture as well. For providing practical training, we have two centers in India, one in Noida (a suburb of New Delhi) and the other in the Himalayan mountains, 400 kilometers north of New Delhi, on the bank of the Ganga. There are short term—one to three week intensive programs—meant to provide you with a living experience of Ayurveda so that you can continue for the rest of your lives with saptakarma, Ayurvedic cooking, spiritual living, and so on.

The main purpose of this network is to spread the message of health care in the world and to bring about a health revolution. I want to make you aware that you are responsible for your own health and you should live your life with the totality of your being. The first priority of life is to safeguard your existence. It is not about just staying alive, it's about your quality of life and living with a happy disposition (prasanchitta).

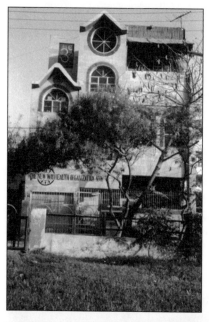

Figure 40. The Noida Center near New Delhi.

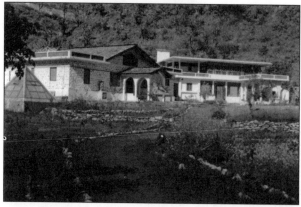

Figure 41. The Himalayan center.

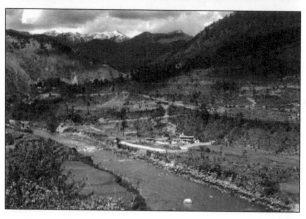

Figure 42. The view from the Himalayan center will totally change your outlook on life.

I hope you will benefit from this ancient Ayurvedic wisdom, and that you will help to spread the Ayurvedic message of holistic living and join me in this crusade for health.

Dr. Vinod Verma
The New Way Health Organization .NOW.
A-130, Sector 26, Noida 201301, UP, India
Telephone 091-11-852 7820; Fax 091-11-855-2368

INDEX

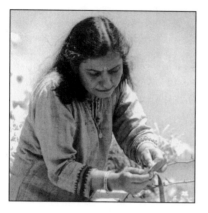

Dr. Vinod Verma assimilated Ayurveda and yoga from her grandmother and father. She earned a Ph.D. in reproductive biology from Panjab University, Chandigarh, and a Ph.D. in neurobiology from the University of Paris (old Sorbonne). She also trained at the prestigious National Institutes of Health, Bethesda, MD, and worked at the Max Planck Institute in Freiburg, Germany. At the peak of her career with a pharmaceutical company in Germany, Dr. Verma realized that our modern Western approach to health is very fragmented, for we are putting all our resources and efforts into curing disease rather than trying to stay healthy. She decided to return to her traditional past, studying Ayurveda and its scriptural tradition from her Ayurvedic guru, Professor Priya Vrat Sharma. She founded the New Way Health Organization in 1987 to spread the message of holistic health care. She now has one center in Noida, near New Delhi, and another in the Himalayan mountains, where she teaches and does research. She is totally dedicated to bringing the home tradition of Ayurveda (her grandmother's tradition) from India to the West, as well as rejuvenating this tradition in her own country. Since she has spent most of her adult life in the West and has traveled all over the world, she understands the various aspects of the culture and traditions of the West, and is able to convey Ayurvedic wisdom to the world with ease. She hosts seminars and lectures, and has been interviewed on TV and radio programs all over the world. She is the author of *Ayurveda for Life* and *Ayurveda as a Way of Life,* both published by Samuel Weiser. She lives part of the year in India, and spends four months a year in Germany and Switzerland.